THE MACRO DIET FOOD-LIST BIBLE:

A Comprehensive Guide to
Eating for Sustainable Weight Loss,
Optimal Health and How to Make the Most of
the Diet with a Comprehensive Meal Plan
and Recipes

MURPHY LAWSON

Copyright © 2023 by **Murphy Lawson**

All rights reserved.

No part of this book may be used or reproduced in any form whatsoever without written permission except in the case of brief quotations in critical articles or reviews.

Printed in the United States of America.

First Edition: **FEBRUARY 2023**

TABLE OF CONTENT

INTRODUCTION 16

UNDERSTANDING THE MACRO DIET 19

The Macro Diet: What Is It? 19

The Macro Diet's Mechanism 21

Determine Your Macronutrient Targets: 21
Monitor Your Macros: 22
Choose Whole, Nutrient-Dense Foods: 22
Make Changes Based on Results: 23

Benefits of the Macro Diet 24

Weight Loss: 24
Increased Muscle Mass: 25
Increased Energy and Focus: 25
Flexibility and Sustainability: 25
Better Overall Health: 26
Customization: 26
Education and Awareness: 27
Better Digestion: 27
Improved Athletic Performance: 28
Support for Specific Dietary Needs: 28

THE THREE MACROS: PROTEIN, CARBOHYDRATES, AND FATS 30

How do macros work? **30**

Carbohydrates: 30
Proteins: 30
Fats: 31

The Role of Protein **32**

Building and repairing tissues: 32
Enzymes and hormones: 33
Immune function: 33
Energy: 33
Appetite control: 34

The Role of Carbohydrates **35**

Energy: 35
Digestive health: 36
Regulation of blood sugar: 36
Sports performance: 36
Macronutrient balancing: 36

The Role of Fats **38**

Energy: 38
Cell membrane structure: 38
Production of hormones: 38
Nutrient absorption: 39
Insulation: 39
Brain and nervous system health: 39

BUILDING YOUR MACRO DIET FOOD LIST 41

Macro-Friendly Foods 41

Lean protein: 41

Whole grains: 42

Fruits and veggies: 42

Healthy fats: 42

Dairy and dairy substitutes: 43

Foods to Avoid 44

Processed Foods: 44

Refined carbohydrates: 44

Sugary beverages: 45

Fried foods: 45

High-fat meats: 45

Dairy with a high fat content: 45

Tips for Grocery Shopping 46

Create a list: 46

Shop the perimeter: 47

Watch for sales: 47

Choose fresh food: 47

Check the labels: 48

Plan your meals: 48

Buy in bulk: 48

MACRO DIET MEAL PLANNING 50

How to Make a Food Plan **50**

Establish your macro objectives: 50
Choose your foods: 50
Plan your meals: 51
Prep your meals: 51
Follow your food plan: 52

Meal Planning Tips and Tricks **53**

Keep it Simple: 53
Plan for leftovers: 53
Employ a meal planning tool: 54
Make a grocery list: 54
Prep ingredients in advance: 54
Be adaptable: 54
Mix & match recipes: 55

Creating Meals Ahead of Time **56**

Choose meals that are simple to prepare: 56
Cook in bulk: 56
Invest in quality containers: 57
Label and date your meals: 57
Have a plan for reheating: 57
Properly store your prepared meals: 58

MEAL PLAN SAMPLES: **59**

WEEK 1 .... **59**

WEEK 2	**63**
WEEK 3	**67**
WEEK 4:	**71**
COOKING TECHNIQUES FOR THE	**76**
MACRO DIET	**76**
Healthy Cooking Techniques	**76**
Choose lean cuts of meat:	76
Use healthy fats:	76
Bake, grill, or broil:	77
Steam your vegetables:	77
Use herbs and spices:	77
Make your own sauces:	77
Macro Diet Cooking Tips and Tricks	**78**
Meal prep:	78
Use a food scale:	79
Track your macros:	79
Experiment with new recipes:	79
Use a variety of spices:	79
Make healthy substitutions:	80
Be mindful of your portions:	80
MACRO DIET RECIPES	**81**
Breakfast Recipes	**81**

1. High-Protein Breakfast Sandwich: 81
2. Blueberry Protein Smoothie: 82
3. Avocado Toast: 83
4. Banana and Peanut Butter Protein Oatmeal: 84
5. Vegetable Frittata: 85
6. Egg and Spinach Breakfast Bowl: 86
7. Banana and Almond Butter Toast: 88
8. Kale and Avocado Toast: 89
9. Avocado Toast with Egg 90
10. Greek Yogurt and Berry Parfait 91
11. Veggie and Cheese Omelette 92
12. Overnight Oats: 93
13. Greek Yogurt Parfait with Berries and Granola 94
14. Scrambled Eggs with Spinach and Feta 96
15. Avocado Toast with Egg and Tomato 97
16. Peanut Butter and Jelly Smoothie 98
17. Greek Yogurt Parfait 99
18. Blueberry Banana Pancakes 100
19. Tofu Scramble 103
20. Spinach and Feta Omelet 105
21. Peanut Butter and Banana Smoothie 106
22. Breakfast Burrito 107
23. Cottage Cheese Pancakes........................ 109

LUNCH RECIPES **111**

1. Grilled Chicken Salad...................................... 111
2. Turkey and Hummus Wrap 112
3. Grilled Veggie and Quinoa Salad............... 112
4. Tuna Salad Lettuce Wraps 113
5. Chicken and Sweet Potato Skillet 114
6. Chicken and Quinoa Salad: 115
7. Tuna and Avocado Wrap: 116
8. Turkey and Hummus Sandwich: 117
9. Veggie Quesadilla: 118
10. Lentil Soup: 119
11. Chickpea Salad Sandwich 120
12. Greek Quinoa Salad 121
13. Turkey and Avocado Wrap 123
14. Quinoa Salad with Roasted Vegetables ... 124
15. Chicken and Broccoli Stir-Fry 125
16. Tuna Salad with Crackers........................... 126
17. Turkey and Hummus Wrap 127
18. Quinoa Salad 128
19. Tuna Salad Lettuce Wraps 130
20. Chickpea and Vegetable Curry 131
21. Salmon and Asparagus Sheet Pan Dinner: 133
22. Pork Chops with Roasted Sweet Potatoes: 134
23. Chicken and Vegetable Stir-Fry: 135

24. Vegetarian Chili: 136
25. Turkey and Zucchini Meatballs: 138
DINNER RECIPES: 139
1. Greek-Style Stuffed Peppers: 139
2. One-Pan Balsamic Chicken and Vegetables: 140
3. Spicy Thai Basil Shrimp: 142
4. Veggie-Packed Quinoa Bowl: 143
5. Baked Salmon with Roasted Vegetables 144
6. Turkey Chili 145
7. Stuffed Bell Peppers 147
8. Grilled Chicken with Vegetables 149
9. Vegetarian Stuffed Bell Peppers 150
10. Baked Salmon with Roasted Broccoli: 152
11. Chicken Fajitas: 153
12. Veggie Burger: 154
13. Turkey and Rice Casserole: 155
14. Grilled Salmon with Sweet Potato Wedges and Asparagus 157
15. Chicken and Vegetable Stir Fry 158
16. Baked Turkey Meatballs with Zucchini Noodles 160
17. Stuffed Bell Peppers 162
18. Grilled Lemon-Herb Chicken with Roasted Vegetables 164

19. Spicy Shrimp Stir-Fry with Rice Noodles 166
20. Baked Salmon with Asparagus and Quinoa 169
21. Lemon Garlic Butter Salmon: 170
21. Quinoa Stuffed Peppers: 172

SNACK RECIPES 174

1. Apple Slices with Almond Butter 174
2. Chocolate Protein Balls 175
3. Greek Yogurt Parfait 175
4. Hummus with Vegetables 176
5. Turkey Roll-Ups 177
6. Fruit and Nut Trail Mix: 178
7. Avocado Toast: 178
8. Hummus and Veggie Sticks: 179
9. Yogurt Parfait: 180
10. Apple and Peanut Butter: 180
11. Baked Sweet Potato Chips 181
12. Chocolate Protein Balls 182
13. Ants on a Log 182
14. Fruit Salad with Yogurt 183
15. Spiced Popcorn 183
16. Greek Yogurt with Honey and Berries 184
17. Spicy Roasted Chickpeas 185
18. Apple Slices with Almond Butter 186
19. Cucumber and Hummus Bites 187

20. Cottage Cheese with Tomato and Basil ... 187
21. Roasted Chickpeas 188
22. Yogurt Parfait 189
23. Apple Slices with Almond Butter 190

DESSERT RECIPES 190

1. Chocolate Protein Mug Cake 190
2. Banana Oat Cookies 192
3. Peanut Butter Protein Balls 193
4. Chocolate Chip Cookies: 194
5. Chocolate Brownies: 196
6. Cheesecake: 197
7. Apple Crisp: 199
Ingredients: 199
8. Chocolate Avocado Pudding 200
9. Protein Brownies 201
Instructions: 202
10. Lemon Chia Seed Muffins 203
11. Chocolate Peanut Butter Protein Balls 204
12. Banana Oat Cookies 205
Instructions: 205
13. Blueberry Protein Muffins 206
14. Chocolate Chia Pudding 208
15. Apple Cinnamon Baked Oatmeal 209
16. Chocolate Protein Brownies 211

17. Peanut Butter Banana Oat Cookies 212
18. Chocolate Chip Banana Bread 213
19. Berry Chia Pudding 215
20. Cinnamon Apple Chips 217
21. Chocolate Chia Pudding: 217
22. Almond Butter and Banana Bites: 218
23. Baked Apple with Cinnamon: 219
24. Chocolate Avocado Pudding: 220
25. Coconut and Berry Chia Seed Pudding: ... 221

STAYING ON TRACK WITH THE MACRO DIET 222

Tips for Dining Out 222

Check the menu in advance: 222
Focus on protein: 222
Watch portion sizes: 223
Avoid creamy sauces and dressings: 223
Choose complex carbohydrates: 223
Don't be afraid to ask for modifications: 224
Avoid sugary drinks: 224

Healthy Snacking Ideas 225

Fresh fruit: 225
Veggies and hummus: 225
Roasted chickpeas: 226
Hard-boiled eggs: 226
Homemade trail mix: 226

Cottage cheese: 226
Rice cakes with avocado and smoked salmon: 227
Edamame: 227
Greek yogurt: 227
Turkey roll-ups: 227

How to Handle Cravings 228

Understand the reason behind the craving: ... 228
Keep healthy snacks on hand: 228
Practice mindfulness: 229
Find healthy alternatives: 229
Allow yourself an occasional treat: 229

Staying Motivated 230

Set Realistic Goals: 230
Find a Support System: 231
Reward Yourself: 231
Keep a Positive Attitude: 232
Track Your Progress: 232
Mix Things Up: 232

CONCLUSION 234

Appendix: Macro Diet Food List Cheat Sheet. 234

Protein: 234
Carbohydrates: 235
Fats: 236

Know your macros: 237
Use portion sizes: 237
Choose whole foods: 238
Schedule your meals: 238
Be adaptable: 238

References **240**

Index 242

INTRODUCTION

I want to start by saying thank you for choosing this book. I hope you found it insightful and helpful.

The Macro Diet Food-List Bible is yours to use. With the aid of the macro diet, you may use this in-depth guide to help you reach your health and weight reduction objectives. The macro diet is a game-changer if you're sick of fad diets that make you feel deprived, hungry, and unhappy. You can provide your body with the nutrition it needs to flourish by concentrating on the proper ratio of macronutrients, including protein, healthy fats, and carbs.

Everything you need to know about the macro diet, including the science behind it and how to make your macro diet food list, is covered in this book. We'll go over the fundamentals of the three macronutrients and show you how to put up scrumptious and nourishing meals. You'll never run out of ideas for wholesome meals that will keep you on track with over 100 macro-friendly recipes.

However, we are aware that maintaining a diet may be difficult, particularly when life interferes. So that you can maintain your diet despite whatever obstacles life throws at you, we've included advice on meal preparation, healthy snacking, and eating out. This book contains something for everyone, whether you're a busy professional, a college student, or a fitness fanatic.

This isn't just another diet book—It's Macro Diet Food-List Bible. It is a thorough resource that will enable you to take charge of your health and accomplish your objectives. Once you give the macro diet a try, we're sure you won't go back. What are you still holding out for? Let's begin the process of making you healthier and happy!

CHAPTER ONE
UNDERSTANDING THE MACRO DIET

The Macro Diet: What Is It?

The balance of macronutrients (proteins, carbs, and fats) in your daily diet is the emphasis of the macro diet, sometimes referred to as flexible dieting. The macro diet places more emphasis on achieving precise macronutrient targets that are suited to your body's needs and objectives than it does on counting calories or avoiding particular meals.

The macro diet involves calculating how many grams of protein, carbs, and fats you should eat each day based on your body weight, amount of exercise, and fitness objectives. Then, as long as they come from full, nutrient-dense sources, you can choose to eat any meals that fall within these macronutrient objectives. With this strategy, you can still achieve your goals while eating more adaptably and sustainably.

Because it ensures that you are giving your body the proper ratio of nutrients it needs to flourish, the macro diet may be a potent tool for weight reduction, muscle building, and general health. The macro diet may be a useful dietary option for many people with the correct information and direction.

The Macro Diet's Mechanism

Instead of calculating calories or avoiding certain foods, the macro diet emphasizes the balance of macronutrients (proteins, carbs, and fats) in your daily diet. Following the macro diet requires the following important steps:

Determine Your Macronutrient Targets: Before beginning the macro diet, you must determine how much protein, carbohydrate, and fat you should eat each day following your body weight, level of exercise, and fitness objectives. You can accomplish this by utilizing an internet calculator or by seeing a dietitian or nutritionist.

Monitor Your Macros: Once you've established your macronutrient goals, you'll need to keep track of how much protein, carbohydrate, and fat you consume each day to make sure you're not exceeding your daily allowances. You may accomplish this by maintaining a food journal or utilizing an app.

Choose Whole, Nutrient-Dense Foods: While the macro diet does not forbid any particular meals, it is crucial to pick full, nutrient-dense foods that fall within your macronutrient objectives. Lean proteins, complex carbs, and healthy fats from foods like fruits, vegetables, whole grains, nuts, seeds, and lean meats should be prioritized to achieve this.

Make Changes Based on Results: Depending on how well you respond to the macro diet, you may need to change your macronutrient objectives. For instance, you might need to change your macronutrient ratios or overall calorie consumption if you're not seeing the desired weight reduction or muscle building.

The macro diet works by giving your body the ideal ratio of macronutrients it requires to function at its best while yet enabling a flexible and sustainable eating pattern. You may reach your health and fitness objectives while taking pleasure in a range of delectable and satiating foods by keeping track of your macronutrients and selecting entire, nutrient-dense foods.

Benefits of the Macro Diet

The macro diet has some potential advantages for people who want to enhance their general health and wellbeing. The following are a few of the primary advantages of the macro diet:

Weight Loss: The macro diet can help you lose weight by ensuring that you're giving your body the proper ratio of macronutrients, which it needs to burn fat and build muscle. You may reduce your calorie intake while still feeling full and satisfied by keeping track of your macronutrients and choosing complete, nutrient-dense foods.

Increased Muscle Mass: If you're trying to put on muscle, the macro diet can help you make sure you're getting enough protein to help your muscles grow. You can assist muscle development and repair after exercise by keeping track of your protein consumption and selecting lean protein sources.

Increased Energy and Focus: The macro diet can help you increase your energy and attention by giving your body the proper ratio of macronutrients. For athletes or people with strenuous careers or lives, this can be very helpful.

Flexibility and Sustainability: The macro diet is adaptable and allows for a large choice of foods, in contrast to many other diets. As a result, it may be simpler to maintain over time and prevent feelings of deprivation or limitation.

Better Overall Health: The macro diet can assist to enhance overall health and lower the risk of chronic illnesses like heart disease, diabetes, and cancer by emphasizing complete, nutrient-dense foods.

Customization: The macro diet may be modified to meet your unique requirements, objectives, and tastes. For instance, you may modify your overall calorie intake to assist weight reduction or muscle building or modify your macronutrient ratios based on your level of exercise.

Education and Awareness: The macro diet aims to raise people's awareness of the importance of macronutrients and how their diet impacts their health. People can become more knowledgeable about the nutritional worth of various meals and make better-educated dietary decisions by keeping track of their macronutrient intake.

Better Digestion: The macro diet can aid in improving digestion and reducing bloating or digestive pain by emphasizing complete, nutrient-dense meals. Furthermore, the high fibre content of many whole meals helps support gut health and regularity.

Improved Athletic Performance: Those who exercise frequently or who are athletes may benefit most from the macro diet. The macro diet can boost recovery after exercise, minimize muscular pain, and increase endurance by giving the body the proper ratio of macronutrients.

Support for Specific Dietary Needs: The macro diet may be tailored to accommodate those who have particular dietary requirements, such as vegetarians or people who are lactose- or gluten-intolerant. A person may still eat enough food to satisfy their nutritional needs while avoiding foods that make them sick or make them allergic by adopting a macronutrient balance that is rich in complete, nutrient-dense meals.

In conclusion, the macro diet has some potential advantages for people who want to enhance their general health and wellbeing. People may optimize their diet for weight reduction, muscle building, better energy and attention, and general health by concentrating on the balance of macronutrients and selecting full, nutrient-dense meals. The macro diet is also versatile and sustainable over the long run since it can be tailored to match unique requirements, tastes, and dietary constraints.

CHAPTER TWO

THE THREE MACROS: PROTEIN, CARBOHYDRATES, AND FATS

How do macros work?

The three primary dietary categories that provide the body energy are known as macronutrients: carbs, proteins, and fats. Every macronutrient has a unique function in the body and contains a range of calories per gram:

Carbohydrates: At 4 calories per gram, carbs are the body's main energy source. Foods including fruits, vegetables, grains, and legumes contain them.

Proteins: Proteins are necessary for the synthesis of enzymes and hormones, as well as for the maintenance and repair of tissues. They are present in meals including meats, fish, eggs, beans, and nuts and offer 4 calories per gram.

Fats: Fats are necessary for the storage of energy, insulation, and the absorption of fat-soluble vitamins. They are present in foods like oils, nuts, seeds, avocados, and fatty seafood, and they have 9 calories per gram.

Those who follow the macro diet keep note of how much of each macronutrient they consume every day to make sure they are getting the proper ratio of nutrients for their requirements and objectives. This might entail keeping track of the grams of each macronutrient ingested throughout the day using a food diary or an app. Individuals may assist with weight reduction, muscle building, and general health and wellbeing by balancing their macronutrient intake.

The Role of Protein

The macronutrient protein, which is needed for numerous basic activities, plays a crucial role in the body. Following are a few of the crucial functions that proteins perform:

Building and repairing tissues: Proteins serve as the building blocks for a variety of bodily tissues, such as muscles, bones, skin, hair, and nails. Protein consumption is crucial for both repairing and growing new tissues.

Enzymes and hormones: A large number of the body's enzymes and hormones are composed of proteins. These molecules are crucial to activities including digestion, metabolism, and the control of bodily functions.

Immune function: Getting adequate protein is crucial for having a robust immune system since many immune cells in the body are composed of proteins.

Energy: While carbs are the body's main source of energy when carbohydrate reserves are low, the body may also use proteins to break down and produce energy.

Appetite control: Protein has been demonstrated to support feelings of fullness and to help limit appetite, which can be beneficial for weight management.

When on the macro diet, people try to eat enough protein to help them achieve their objectives, such as boosting weight reduction or muscle growth. The quantity of protein required might change based on characteristics including age, sex, weight, and degree of exercise. On the macro diet, the recommended protein consumption ranges from moderate to high, with some programs calling for 1 gram of protein per pound of body weight. People may support muscle growth and repair, control appetite, and advance general health and wellbeing by making protein a priority in their diets.

The Role of Carbohydrates

An essential macronutrient, carbohydrates have many vital functions in the body. Following are a few of the primary roles that carbs play:

Energy: Glucose, which the body uses as fuel, is produced by carbohydrates and is the body's main source of energy. The efficient functioning of the brain, neurological system, and red blood cells depends on glucose.

Digestive health: Some forms of carbs, such as fibre, are crucial for digestion and can control bowel motions.

Regulation of blood sugar: The body has systems in place to control blood sugar levels, which can be affected by consuming carbs. A hormone called insulin is produced in reaction to carbs and aids in controlling blood sugar levels.

Sports performance: Carbohydrates are crucial for athletes and anyone who exercise because they give the body a rapid source of energy when exercising.

Macronutrient balancing: It's crucial for general health and can help with weight control to balance carbohydrate consumption with that of protein and fat.

Those who follow the macro diet keep track of their carbohydrate consumption to make sure they are obtaining the proper nutrients for their objectives and needs. This may entail restricting some sources of carbs, including refined sugars and processed meals while giving whole grains, fruits, and vegetables the top priority. Individuals may maintain energy levels, control blood sugar, and advance general health and wellbeing by maximizing their carbohydrate consumption.

The Role of Fats

Lipids, another name for fats, are essential macronutrients that the body uses for many purposes. Following are a few of the primary uses for fats:

Energy: The body uses fats as a source of energy, and they deliver more than twice as much as protein or carbs.

Cell membrane structure: Fats are a crucial part of cell membrane structure and are involved in keeping cells' structural integrity and functionality.

Production of hormones: Fats are used in the creation of several hormones, including estrogen and testosterone.

Nutrient absorption: Fats are required for the absorption of several fat-soluble vitamins, including vitamins A, D, E, and K.

Insulation: Fats may shield and defend the body from climatic changes and physical harm.

Brain and nervous system health: Fats are essential for the health of the brain and nervous system because they make up the myelin sheath, which protects nerve cells.

Those who follow the macro diet try to eat a variety of fats, such as saturated, monounsaturated, and polyunsaturated fats, in moderation. This may entail increasing the consumption of nutritious fat sources such as nuts, seeds, avocados, and fatty fish while reducing the consumption of bad ones like processed meals and fried foods. Individuals may promote their general health and well-being, including hormone synthesis, nutrition absorption, and brain and nervous system function, by maximizing their consumption of fats.

CHAPTER THREE
BUILDING YOUR MACRO DIET FOOD LIST

Macro-Friendly Foods

Foods that are macro-friendly improve general health and wellbeing by being nutrient-dense and offering a balance of macronutrients. These are some examples of foods that are macro-friendly:

Lean protein: which is essential for repairing and constructing muscle tissue among other things, may be found in a variety of foods including chicken, turkey, fish, tofu, tempeh, and legumes.

Whole grains: Complex carbs in whole grains, such as brown rice, quinoa, and oats, are absorbed slowly and help control blood sugar levels while prolonging satiety.

Fruits and veggies: Fruits and vegetables are rich in vitamins, minerals, fibre, and other nutrients. Moreover, they offer carbs, a vital source of energy.

Healthy fats: Nuts, seeds, avocados, and fatty fish are examples of sources of healthy fats. These foods are crucial for maintaining hormone synthesis, nutrition absorption, and brain and nervous system health.

Dairy and dairy substitutes: Low-fat or fat-free dairy products, such as milk, yoghurt, and cheese, can be a good source of calcium, protein, and carbs. Nutrient-rich dairy substitutes like soy or almond milk can also be found.

Aiming to balance their intake of these macro-friendly foods, while restricting or eliminating processed meals, refined sugars, and harmful fats is the goal of the macro diet. Blood sugar levels can be managed, weight can be maintained, and general health and wellbeing can be supported.

Foods to Avoid

Because of their propensity to be rich in calories, bad fats, and added sugars, some food groups are often restricted or avoided when adhering to the macro diet. In the macro diet, the following items should be avoided or limited:

Processed Foods: Foods that have been processed frequently include a lot of calories, bad fats, and added sweets, such as chips, cookies, and frozen meals.

Refined carbohydrates: Meals like white bread, spaghetti, and pastries made from refined flour tend to be poor in nutrients and can cause blood sugar levels to rise.

Sugary beverages: Sugary beverages, including soda, juice, and energy drinks, can be a significant source of extra sugar and empty calories.

Fried foods: Fried meals are frequently heavy in harmful fats and calories, such as fried chicken and french fries.

High-fat meats: Meats like bacon, sausage, and beef can contain a lot of calories and dangerous saturated fats.

Dairy with a high-fat content: Dairy products with a high-fat content, including whole milk, cream, and butter, also have a high-calorie content and a high saturated fat content.

Even though you don't have to fully cut out these foods from your diet, doing so can support weight management, control blood sugar levels, and advance general health and wellbeing. People may develop a lasting, healthy eating routine that supports their goals by concentrating on a balance of macro-friendly foods.

Tips for Grocery Shopping

A key component of properly implementing the macro diet is grocery shopping. Here are some pointers to help you have more effective grocery shopping trips:

Create a list: List the macro-friendly foods you must purchase before going to the supermarket. This can aid in maintaining attention and preventing impulsive purchases.

Shop the perimeter: Freshest and healthiest goods, such as fruits, vegetables, lean meats, and dairy products, are frequently found in the grocery store's outside aisles. Spend most of your time here.

Watch for sales: When you go shopping, seek discounts on macro-friendly foods like lean meats, healthy grains, and fresh fruit by checking the weekly sales flyers.

Choose fresh food: Compared to their canned or frozen equivalents, fresh fruits, vegetables, and meats are often healthier and less processed.

Check the labels: before buying packaged foods to be sure there aren't any bad fats, sugar additives, or other components that might not be macro-friendly.

Plan your meals: If you intend to prepare your meals in advance for the entire week, choose ingredients that can be prepared quickly and in big quantities, such as brown rice, chicken breasts, and mixed vegetables.

Buy in bulk: Purchase macro-friendly foods in bulk, such as whole grains, nuts, and seeds, if you have the storage space. This can help you save money and cut down on the number of visits you need to go to the store.

You may make it simpler to keep to the macro diet and reach your health and fitness objectives by using this grocery shopping advice.

CHAPTER FOUR
MACRO DIET MEAL PLANNING

How to Make a Food Plan

A key component of effectively implementing the macro diet is making a food plan. The following steps will assist you in creating a macro-friendly diet plan:

Establish your macro objectives: Based on your age, gender, weight, and degree of exercise, you should first establish your daily macro goals. You may choose your daily macro goals with the aid of online tools and mobile applications.

Choose your foods: If you are aware of your macro objectives, pick meals that will assist you in achieving them. Foods high in protein, complex carbs, and healthy fats should be your main priority. Lean meats, fish, whole grains, fruits, vegetables, nuts, and seeds are a few examples of macro-friendly foods.

Plan your meals: Create a weekly menu using a meal planning tool or template. Be sure to balance your macros throughout the day by including breakfast, lunch, supper, and snacks.

Prep your meals: Once you've established a meal plan, it's time to prepare your meals. This might entail cutting veggies, preparing smoothie components, or cooking and portioning meals in advance. Meal preparation can help you save time and make it simpler to follow your weekly macros.

Follow your food plan: but keep an eye on your progress and make any necessary adjustments. To help you reach your macro objectives, you might need to make adjustments to your meal plan over time.

You may make a macro-friendly diet plan that will help you reach your fitness and health objectives by using the strategies listed below. The macro diet may become a sustainable and pleasurable aspect of living a healthy lifestyle with time and effort.

Meal Planning Tips and Tricks

Even though meal preparation can be difficult, there are ways to make it simpler and more fun. Here are some advice and strategies for the macro diet's meal preparation:

Keep it Simple: When you first start, make your food plan straightforward. Choose recipes that call for simple, everyday items. You can explore trickier recipes as you get more at ease.

Plan for leftovers: when you prepare they can be utilized as leftovers as part of your planning for leftovers. When you are pressed for time later in the week, this will save you time and effort.

Employ a meal planning tool: You may plan your meals and determine your macros using a variety of online resources, including websites and apps.

Make a grocery list: Create a list of the items you'll need for the week's worth of meals before you go shopping. You'll save time and prevent making impulsive purchases as a result.

Prep ingredients in advance: Spend some time preparing the items in advance, for as by cutting the veggies or marinating the meats. This will make cooking during the week simpler and faster.

Be adaptable: Don't be hesitant to alter your eating plan as necessary. Replace a recipe that doesn't work for you with one that does and that still fits your macros.

Mix & match recipes: To be able to vary your meals throughout the week, look for recipes that call for comparable items. For instance, a roasted chicken can be utilized in a salad for lunch the following day after being served for dinner the previous night.

You may make meal planning simpler and more fun by using the advice provided here. Being prepared, organized, and adaptable is crucial. You'll master macro meal planning with some training.

Creating Meals Ahead of Time

Making meals ahead of time is a terrific way to save time and guarantee that you always have wholesome, macro-friendly meals on hand. Here are some pointers for meal preparation in advance:

Choose meals that are simple to prepare: Casseroles, soups, and salads are some examples of recipes that may be prepared ahead of time. Choose dishes that can be prepared in big quantities and kept in the refrigerator or freezer.

Cook in bulk: Make a lot of food when you're cooking so that there are meals left over. When you are pressed for time later in the week, this will save you time and effort.

Invest in quality containers: Spend money on high-quality containers that may be used for both storage and reheating. Glass containers with snap-on lids are an excellent choice since they are robust and functional in both the oven and microwave.

Label and date your meals: before putting them in the refrigerator or freezer. You can keep track of what you have and when it was created by doing this.

Have a plan for reheating: When you're prepared to consume your prepared meals, have a strategy for warming them. While some meals may be consumed cold, some might require reheating in the microwave or oven.

Properly store your prepared meals: In the refrigerator or freezer, depending on when you'll be eating them. Meals that will be consumed later on in the week or month can be stored in the freezer while meals that will be consumed within a few days can be kept in the refrigerator.

You can save time and make sure you always have wholesome, macro-friendly meals on hand by preparing your meals in advance. You may stick to your macro diet by making meal preparation a regular part of your routine with a little planning and preparation.

MEAL PLAN SAMPLES:

here's a Four-week meal plan for the Macro Diet:

WEEK 1

Monday

Breakfast: Greek yoghurt parfait with mixed berries, chia seeds, and honey

Snack: Apple slices with almond butter

Lunch: Chicken and vegetable stir-fry with brown rice

Snack: Protein smoothie with spinach, banana, peanut butter, and almond milk

Dinner: Grilled salmon with asparagus and roasted sweet potatoes

Tuesday

Breakfast: Scrambled eggs with spinach, mushrooms, and avocado

Snack: Carrots and hummus

Lunch: Turkey and Swiss cheese wrap with mixed greens and whole wheat tortilla

Snack: Plain Greek yoghurt with sliced peaches and honey

Dinner: Turkey meatballs with zucchini noodles and marinara sauce

Wednesday

Breakfast: Protein pancakes with mixed berries and pure maple syrup

Snack: String cheese with grapes

Lunch: Grilled chicken salad with mixed greens, cherry tomatoes, cucumber, and balsamic vinaigrette

Snack: Cottage cheese with pineapple chunks

Dinner: Beef and broccoli stir-fried with brown rice

Thursday

Breakfast: Breakfast burrito with scrambled eggs, black beans, avocado, and salsa

Snack: Whole grain crackers with low-fat cheese

Lunch: Tuna salad with mixed greens and whole wheat crackers

Snack: Mixed berries with whipped cream

Dinner: Baked chicken breast with roasted Brussels sprouts and quinoa

Friday

Breakfast: Smoothie bowl with Greek yoghurt, mixed berries, chia seeds, and granola

Snack: Hard-boiled eggs with a sprinkle of sea salt

Lunch: Grilled chicken sandwich with mixed greens and whole wheat bread

Snack: Peanut butter and apple slices

Dinner: Shrimp and vegetable stir-fry with brown rice

Saturday

Breakfast: Scrambled eggs with spinach and tomato slices, whole wheat toast

Snack: Mixed nuts with dried cranberries

Lunch: Whole grain wrap with roasted turkey, lettuce, and tomato slices

Snack: Greek yoghurt with sliced banana and honey

Dinner: Beef fajitas with mixed peppers, onions, and whole wheat tortillas

Sunday

Breakfast: Omelette with mushrooms, spinach, and feta cheese

Snack: Cottage cheese with cherry tomatoes

Lunch: Grilled salmon salad with mixed greens, cucumber, and tomato

Snack: Rice cakes with almond butter and banana slices

Dinner: Grilled chicken kebabs with mixed peppers, onions, and brown rice.

WEEK 2

Monday:

Breakfast: Oatmeal with almond milk, banana, and walnuts

Lunch: Grilled chicken with quinoa, steamed broccoli, and a side salad

Snack: Greek yoghurt with fresh berries

Dinner: Grilled salmon with roasted sweet potatoes and asparagus

Tuesday:

Breakfast: Avocado toast with two boiled eggs

Lunch: Quinoa and black bean salad with avocado, tomato, and cilantro

Snack: Apple slices with almond butter

Dinner: Baked cod with roasted Brussels sprouts and carrots

Wednesday:

Breakfast: Smoothie bowl with almond milk, banana, spinach, and chia seeds

Lunch: Lentil soup with a side of brown rice

Snack: Celery sticks with hummus

Dinner: Baked chicken with couscous and steamed green beans

Thursday:

Breakfast: Whole grain toast with almond butter and sliced banana

Lunch: Tuna salad with quinoa and roasted vegetables

Snack: Greek yoghurt with berries

Dinner: Grilled turkey with sweet potatoes and roasted zucchini

Friday:

Breakfast: Omelet with vegetables and ricotta cheese

Lunch: Grilled turkey and veggie wrap

Snack: Almonds and an apple

Dinner: Grilled salmon with steamed brown rice and roasted Brussels sprouts

Saturday:

Breakfast: Oatmeal with almond milk and sliced almonds

Lunch: Quinoa salad with grilled chicken

Snack: Hummus and vegetable sticks

Dinner: Baked cod with roasted sweet potatoes and asparagus

Sunday:

Breakfast: Smoothie bowl with almond milk, banana, spinach, and chia seeds

Lunch: Lentil soup with a side of brown rice

Snack: Apple slices with almond butter

Dinner: Baked chicken with couscous and steamed green beans.

WEEK 3

Monday

Breakfast: Greek yoghurt with mixed berries and chopped nuts

Lunch: Tuna salad with mixed greens, cherry tomatoes, and avocado

Snack: Carrots and hummus

Dinner: Baked chicken breast with roasted sweet potatoes and sautéed green beans

Tuesday

Breakfast: Spinach and mushroom omelette with whole-grain toast

Lunch: Quinoa and black bean salad with chopped bell pepper, cucumber, and feta cheese

Snack: Apple slices with almond butter

Dinner: Turkey chilli with mixed vegetables and a side of brown rice

Wednesday

Breakfast: Protein smoothie with mixed frozen berries, spinach, and protein powder

Lunch: Grilled chicken breast with mixed vegetables and a side of quinoa

Snack: Plain Greek yoghurt with honey and chopped nuts

Dinner: Grilled salmon with roasted Brussels sprouts and a side of mashed sweet potatoes

Thursday

Breakfast: Egg and cheese breakfast sandwich with whole grain English muffin

Lunch: Chicken and vegetable stir-fry with brown rice

Snack: Baby carrots with hummus

Dinner: Ground turkey tacos with mixed vegetables and a side of black beans

Friday

Breakfast: Protein pancakes with mixed berries and a side of turkey bacon

Lunch: Grilled chicken Caesar salad with whole grain croutons and shaved Parmesan

Snack: Fresh fruit salad with mixed berries, sliced kiwi, and chopped pineapple

Dinner: Grilled flank steak with mixed vegetables and a side of quinoa

Saturday

Breakfast: Protein smoothie with mixed frozen berries, spinach, and protein powder

Lunch: Turkey and cheese sandwich with mixed greens, tomato, and avocado

Snack: Trail mix with mixed nuts and dried fruit

Dinner: Grilled shrimp skewers with mixed vegetables and a side of brown rice

Sunday

Breakfast: Egg and cheese breakfast sandwich with whole grain English muffin

Lunch: Baked sweet potato topped with black beans, diced avocado, and salsa

Snack: Low-fat string cheese with grapes

Dinner: Grilled chicken breast with roasted root vegetables and a side of quinoa

WEEK 4:

Monday

Breakfast: Greek yoghurt with mixed berries, honey, and chopped almonds

Snack: Hard-boiled egg

Lunch: Grilled chicken breast with roasted sweet potato and steamed broccoli

Snack: Apple slices with almond butter

Dinner: Baked salmon with quinoa and roasted asparagus

Tuesday

Breakfast: Scrambled eggs with spinach and sliced avocado

Snack: Sliced bell peppers with hummus

Lunch: Turkey chilli with brown rice and mixed greens

Snack: Banana with almond butter

Dinner: Grilled sirloin steak with roasted Brussels sprouts and sweet potato wedges

Wednesday

Breakfast: Omelet with mushrooms, spinach, and feta cheese

Snack: Low-fat cottage cheese with pineapple chunks

Lunch: Grilled shrimp with mixed greens and quinoa salad

Snack: Carrot sticks with hummus

Dinner: Baked chicken thighs with roasted carrots and cauliflower

Thursday

Breakfast: Overnight oats with almond milk, mixed berries, and chia seeds

Snack: Apple slices with peanut butter

Lunch: Grilled chicken salad with mixed greens, cherry tomatoes, and avocado

Snack: Baby carrots with hummus

Dinner: Baked tilapia with roasted zucchini and brown rice

Friday

Breakfast: Low-fat cottage cheese with sliced peaches and chopped walnuts

Snack: Hard-boiled egg

Lunch: Turkey and avocado wrap with mixed greens

Snack: Sliced cucumbers with hummus

Dinner: Grilled pork chops with roasted sweet potatoes and green beans

Saturday

Breakfast: Greek yoghurt with mixed berries, honey, and chopped almonds
Snack: Apple slices with almond butter
Lunch: Grilled chicken breast with mixed greens and quinoa salad
Snack: Sliced bell peppers with hummus
Dinner: Baked salmon with roasted asparagus and brown rice

Sunday

Breakfast: Scrambled eggs with mushrooms and sliced avocado
Snack: Low-fat cottage cheese with pineapple chunks
Lunch: Turkey chilli with mixed greens and brown rice
Snack: Banana with almond butter

Dinner: Grilled sirloin steak with roasted Brussels sprouts and sweet potato wedges

CHAPTER FIVE
COOKING TECHNIQUES FOR THE MACRO DIET

Healthy Cooking Techniques

Healthy cooking techniques can help you make macro-friendly meals that are delicious and nutritious. Here are some tips for healthy cooking:

Choose lean cuts of meat: Choose lean cuts of meat that are low in fat, such as chicken breast, turkey breast, or sirloin steak.

Use healthy fats: Use healthy fats, such as olive oil, avocado oil, or coconut oil, in moderation. Avoid cooking with butter or margarine.

Bake, grill, or broil: Use baking, grilling, or broiling to cook your meat and vegetables. These methods allow you to cook your food without adding extra fat or calories.

Steam your vegetables: Steaming is a healthy way to cook your vegetables, as it preserves their nutrients and flavour.

Use herbs and spices: Use herbs and spices to add flavour to your meals, instead of relying on salt and sugar.

Make your sauces: Avoid using pre-made sauces and dressings, which can be high in fat and calories. Instead, make your sauces using healthy ingredients, such as yoghurt, tomatoes, or garlic.

By using these healthy cooking techniques, you can make macro-friendly meals that are both delicious and nutritious. Experiment with different recipes and ingredients to find the ones that work best for you and your taste preferences.

Macro Diet Cooking Tips and Tricks

Cooking for the macro diet requires a bit of planning and creativity, but with the right tips and tricks, you can make healthy and delicious meals. Here are some macro diet cooking tips:

Meal prep: Plan your meals and meal prep for the week. This will save you time and ensure that you have healthy meals ready to eat.

Use a food scale: Weigh your ingredients with a food scale to ensure that you are getting the right portions of protein, carbohydrates, and fats.

Track your macros: Use a macro-tracking app or journal to track your daily intake of protein, carbohydrates, and fats.

Experiment with new recipes: Try new recipes that fit your macros to avoid getting bored with your meals. There are plenty of macro-friendly recipes online.

Use a variety of spices: Use spices and herbs to add flavour to your meals without adding extra calories or salt.

Make healthy substitutions: Make healthy substitutions in your favourite recipes, such as using Greek yoghurt instead of sour cream or almond flour instead of wheat flour.

Be mindful of your portions: Pay attention to your portion sizes to avoid overeating and going over your macros.

By using these cooking tips and tricks, you can create delicious and satisfying meals that meet your macro requirements. Remember, the key to success is planning, tracking, and experimenting with new recipes.

CHAPTER SIX
MACRO DIET RECIPES

Breakfast Recipes

Here are macro-friendly breakfast recipes with a list of ingredients and instructions:

1. High-Protein Breakfast Sandwich:

Ingredients:

1 whole-grain English muffin

2 egg whites

1 slice of reduced-fat cheese

1 slice of lean ham or turkey

Salt and pepper to taste

Instructions:

Preheat a non-stick pan over medium heat.

Whisk the egg whites with salt and pepper and pour them into the pan.

Once the egg whites are set, flip them over and place the cheese on top.

Toast the English muffin and layer the ham or turkey on the bottom half.

Add the egg and cheese on top and serve.

2. Blueberry Protein Smoothie:

Ingredients:

1 cup of unsweetened almond milk

1 scoop of vanilla whey protein powder

1/2 cup of frozen blueberries

1 tablespoon of almond butter

1 teaspoon of honey

Instructions:

Add all the ingredients to a blender and blend until smooth.

If the consistency is too thick, add more almond milk until it reaches the desired consistency.

Pour into a glass and enjoy.

3. Avocado Toast:

Ingredients:

1 slice of whole-grain bread

1/2 of an avocado

1 small tomato, sliced

Salt and pepper to taste

Instructions:

Toast the bread.

Mash the avocado with salt and pepper and spread it on the toast.

Top with sliced tomato and serve.

4. Banana and Peanut Butter Protein Oatmeal:

Ingredients:

1/2 cup of rolled oats

1 cup of water

1 scoop of vanilla whey protein powder

1/2 banana, sliced

1 tablespoon of peanut butter

Cinnamon to taste

Instructions:

Add the rolled oats and water to a microwave-safe bowl and microwave for 2-3 minutes, or until cooked.

Stir in the protein powder and cinnamon.

Top with sliced banana and peanut butter.

5. Vegetable Frittata:

Ingredients:
4 eggs
1/4 cup of unsweetened almond milk
1/2 cup of chopped vegetables (e.g., spinach, mushrooms, onions)
Salt and pepper to taste

Instructions:

Preheat the oven to 350°F.

Whisk the eggs, almond milk, salt, and pepper in a bowl.

Add the chopped vegetables to an oven-safe skillet and sauté over medium heat.

Pour the egg mixture over the vegetables and stir to combine.

Transfer the skillet to the oven and bake for 10-15 minutes or until the eggs are set. Slice and serve.

6. Egg and Spinach Breakfast Bowl:

Ingredients:
- 2 eggs
- 2 cups of spinach
- 1/2 cup of diced bell peppers

- 2 tablespoons of olive oil

- Salt and pepper to taste

Instructions:

1. Heat the olive oil in a skillet over medium heat.

2. Add the diced bell peppers and sauté for 3-4 minutes.

3. Add the spinach and sauté for another 3-4 minutes, or until the spinach has wilted.

4. Crack the eggs into the skillet and cook for 3-4 minutes, or until the whites are firm and the yolks are cooked to your liking.

5. Season with salt and pepper to taste.

6. Serve in a bowl and enjoy!

7. Banana and Almond Butter Toast:

Ingredients:
- 2 slices of whole wheat toast
- 2 tablespoons of almond butter
- 1 banana, sliced
- 1 tablespoon of honey

Instructions:
1. Toast the two slices of whole wheat toast until golden brown.
2. Spread the almond butter onto the toast.
3. Top the toast with the sliced banana.
4. Drizzle the honey over
5. Enjoy!

8. Kale and Avocado Toast:

Ingredients:
- 2 slices of whole wheat toast
- 1/2 an avocado, mashed
- 1/2 cup of kale, chopped
- 2 tablespoons of olive oil
- Salt and pepper to taste

Instructions:
1. Toast the two slices of whole wheat toast until golden brown.
2. Spread the mashed avocado onto the toast.
3. Top the toast with the chopped kale.
4. Drizzle the olive oil over the toast and season with salt and pepper to taste.
5. Enjoy!

9. Avocado Toast with Egg

Ingredients:

2 slices whole grain bread

1 ripe avocado

2 eggs

Salt and pepper to taste

Instructions:

Toast the bread to your desired level of crispness.

Mash the avocado in a small bowl and season with salt and pepper to taste.

In a skillet over medium heat, cook the eggs to your preferred level of doneness (sunny-side up or scrambled).

Spread the mashed avocado onto the toasted bread and top with the cooked egg. Serve immediately.

10. Greek Yogurt and Berry Parfait

Ingredients:

1 cup Greek yoghurt

1/2 cup mixed berries (strawberries, blueberries, raspberries)

1/4 cup granola

1 tsp honey

Instructions:

In a small bowl, mix the Greek yoghurt and honey.

In a separate bowl, layer the mixed berries and granola.

Top the berry and granola mixture with the Greek yoghurt mixture.

Serve immediately.

11. Veggie and Cheese Omelette

Ingredients:

2 eggs

1/4 cup chopped bell pepper

1/4 cup chopped onion

1/4 cup shredded cheddar cheese

Salt and pepper to taste

1 tsp olive oil

Instructions:

In a small bowl, whisk the eggs together with salt and pepper to taste.

Heat the olive oil in a small skillet over medium heat.

Add the chopped bell pepper and onion to the skillet and sauté for 2-3 minutes, until the vegetables are softened.

Pour the eggs into the skillet, tilting the pan to distribute the eggs evenly.

Allow the eggs to cook for 2-3 minutes, then sprinkle the shredded cheddar cheese over the omelette.

Use a spatula to fold the omelette in half, then slide it onto a plate.

Serve immediately.

12. Overnight Oats:

Ingredients:
- 1/2 cup of old-fashioned oats
- 1/2 cup of unsweetened almond milk

- 1/2 teaspoon of cinnamon
- 1 tablespoon of chia seeds
- 1 tablespoon of honey
- 1/4 cup of blueberries

Instructions:

1. In a jar or container, add the oats, almond milk, cinnamon, chia seeds, and honey and mix to combine.
2. Cover the jar or container and place it in the refrigerator overnight.
3. In the morning, stir in the blueberries.
4. Enjoy!

13. Greek Yogurt Parfait with Berries and Granola

Ingredients:

1 cup plain nonfat Greek yoghurt

1/2 cup mixed berries (such as raspberries, blueberries, and strawberries)

1/4 cup granola

1 tablespoon honey

Instructions:

In a small bowl, mix the Greek yoghurt and honey.

In a glass or bowl, layer the yoghurt mixture, berries, and granola.

Repeat the layers until all the ingredients are used up.

Serve immediately.

14. Scrambled Eggs with Spinach and Feta

Ingredients:

2 large eggs

1/4 cup baby spinach, chopped

1 tablespoon crumbled feta cheese

1/2 tablespoon olive oil

Salt and pepper, to taste

Instructions:

In a small bowl, whisk together the eggs, salt, and pepper.

In a nonstick skillet over medium heat, heat the olive oil.

Add the spinach to the skillet and cook until wilted, stirring occasionally.

Pour the egg mixture into the skillet and cook, stirring occasionally, until the eggs are set.

Sprinkle the feta cheese over the eggs and serve hot.

15. Avocado Toast with Egg and Tomato

Ingredients:

1 slice of whole-grain bread, toasted

1/2 ripe avocado, mashed

1 large egg

1/4 cup cherry tomatoes, halved

1/2 tablespoon olive oil

Salt and pepper, to taste

Instructions:

Spread the mashed avocado on the toasted bread.

In a nonstick skillet over medium heat, heat the olive oil.

Crack the egg into the skillet and cook to your desired level of doneness, seasoning with salt and pepper.

Place the cooked egg on top of the avocado toast.

Serve with cherry tomatoes on the side.

16. Peanut Butter and Jelly Smoothie

Ingredients:

1 ripe banana

1/2 cup frozen mixed berries

1/2 cup unsweetened almond milk

2 tablespoons natural peanut butter

1 tablespoon honey

Instructions:

In a blender, combine the banana, mixed berries, almond milk, peanut butter, and honey.

Blend until smooth and creamy.

Pour into a glass and serve immediately.

17. Greek Yogurt Parfait

Ingredients:

1 cup plain Greek yoghurt

1/2 cup fresh berries (strawberries, blueberries, or raspberries)

1/4 cup granola

1 tbsp honey

Instructions:

In a glass or a bowl, add a layer of Greek yoghurt.

Add a layer of fresh berries on top of the yoghurt.

Sprinkle a layer of granola over the berries.

Drizzle honey over the granola.

Repeat layers until you reach the top.

Enjoy!

18. Blueberry Banana Pancakes

Ingredients:

1 cup all-purpose flour

2 tbsp granulated sugar

2 tsp baking powder

1/4 tsp salt

1 ripe banana, mashed

1 egg

1 cup milk

1/2 cup fresh blueberries

Butter or oil for cooking

Instructions:

In a large bowl, whisk together the flour, sugar, baking powder, and salt.

In a separate bowl, whisk together the mashed banana, egg, and milk until well combined.

Add the wet ingredients to the dry ingredients and mix until just combined.

Fold in the blueberries.

Heat a non-stick skillet over medium-high heat.

Melt a small amount of butter or oil in the skillet.

Scoop about 1/4 cup of batter per pancake onto the skillet.

Cook until bubbles appear on the surface and the edges start to dry about 2-3 minutes.

Flip the pancake and cook for an additional 1-2 minutes until golden brown.

Repeat with the remaining batter.

Serve warm with additional blueberries and maple syrup.

19. Tofu Scramble

Ingredients:

1 block firm tofu, drained and crumbled
1 tbsp olive oil
1/2 small onion, chopped
1/2 red bell pepper, chopped
1/2 tsp garlic powder
1/2 tsp cumin
1/2 tsp turmeric
Salt and pepper to taste

Instructions:

Heat the olive oil in a large skillet over medium heat.

Add the chopped onion and red bell pepper and sauté until soft, about 5 minutes.

Add the crumbled tofu to the skillet and stir to combine.

Add the garlic powder, cumin, turmeric, salt, and pepper and stir to evenly distribute the spices.

Cook for an additional 5-7 minutes, stirring occasionally until the tofu is heated through and slightly browned.

Serve hot.

20. Spinach and Feta Omelet

Ingredients:

2 eggs

1/2 cup fresh spinach

1/4 cup crumbled feta cheese

1/4 teaspoon garlic powder

Salt and pepper to taste

1 teaspoon olive oil

Instructions:

Whisk the eggs in a bowl and add salt, pepper, and garlic powder.

Heat olive oil in a non-stick pan over medium heat.

Add fresh spinach and sauté until wilted.

Add the egg mixture to the pan and swirl to cover the bottom.

Sprinkle the feta cheese on top of the egg mixture.

Use a spatula to gently fold the omelette in half and cook until the cheese is melted and the egg is set.

Serve hot.

21. Peanut Butter and Banana Smoothie

Ingredients:

1 banana

1 cup unsweetened almond milk

2 tablespoons natural peanut butter

1 scoop vanilla protein powder

1/4 teaspoon ground cinnamon

1 cup ice cubes

Instructions:

Add all ingredients to a blender and blend until smooth.

Serve immediately.

22. Breakfast Burrito

Ingredients:

2 eggs, beaten

1/4 cup black beans, drained and rinsed

1/4 cup shredded cheddar cheese

1/4 cup diced tomatoes

2 tablespoons chopped cilantro

1 whole wheat tortilla

Instructions:

Heat a non-stick pan over medium heat and spray with cooking spray.

Add the beaten eggs to the pan and scramble until set.

Warm the tortilla in the microwave for 10-15 seconds.

Add the scrambled eggs, black beans, cheddar cheese, diced tomatoes, and cilantro to the centre of the tortilla.

Fold the sides of the tortilla inward, then roll up from the bottom to form a burrito.

Serve hot.

23. Cottage Cheese Pancakes

Ingredients:

1 cup low-fat cottage cheese

1/2 cup rolled oats

2 eggs

1 teaspoon vanilla extract

1/4 teaspoon baking powder

1/4 teaspoon salt

1 tablespoon butter, melted

Instructions:

Add all ingredients to a blender and blend until smooth.

Heat a non-stick pan over medium heat and spray with cooking spray.

Pour 1/4 cup of the batter into the pan and cook for 2-3 minutes on each side, until golden brown.

Repeat with the remaining batter.

Serve hot with your favourite toppings.

These recipes are just a few examples of macro-friendly breakfast options. Experiment with different ingredients and recipes to find the ones that work best for you and your taste preferences. Remember to track your macros to ensure that you are meeting your daily requirements.

LUNCH RECIPES

here are 20 Plus Lunch recipes:

1. Grilled Chicken Salad

4 oz grilled chicken breast, sliced

2 cups mixed greens

1/2 avocado, diced

1/4 cup cherry tomatoes, halved

1/4 cup sliced cucumber

2 tbsp balsamic vinaigrette

Instructions:

Arrange mixed greens in a bowl. Top with grilled chicken, avocado, cherry tomatoes, and sliced cucumber. Drizzle with balsamic vinaigrette.

2. Turkey and Hummus Wrap

1 whole wheat tortilla

3 oz deli turkey

2 tbsp hummus

1/4 cup spinach

1/4 cup diced bell peppers

1/4 cup diced cucumber

Instructions:

Spread hummus on the tortilla. Top with turkey, spinach, bell peppers, and cucumber. Roll up and slice in half.

3. Grilled Veggie and Quinoa Salad

1/2 cup quinoa

1/4 cup diced zucchini

1/4 cup diced eggplant

1/4 cup diced red bell pepper

1/4 cup diced red onion

1 tbsp olive oil

1 tbsp balsamic vinegar

1 tbsp chopped fresh parsley

Instructions:

Cook quinoa according to package instructions. Preheat the grill to medium-high heat. Toss vegetables with olive oil and grill until tender. In a large bowl, mix quinoa, grilled vegetables, balsamic vinegar, and chopped parsley.

4. Tuna Salad Lettuce Wraps

1 can of tuna in water, drained

1 tbsp mayo

1/4 cup diced celery

1/4 cup diced red onion

Salt and pepper, to taste

4 lettuce leaves

Instructions:

In a small bowl, mix tuna, mayo, celery, red onion, salt, and pepper. Spoon tuna salad onto each lettuce leaf, then wrap and serve.

5. Chicken and Sweet Potato Skillet

4 oz boneless, skinless chicken breast, cubed

1 medium sweet potato, peeled and diced

1/4 cup diced red onion

1/4 cup diced green bell pepper

1 tbsp olive oil

1/2 tsp smoked paprika

1/4 tsp garlic powder

Salt and pepper, to taste

Instructions:

Heat olive oil in a skillet over medium heat. Add chicken and cook until browned. Add sweet potato, red onion, and green bell pepper to the skillet. Season with smoked paprika, garlic powder, salt, and pepper. Cook until sweet potato is tender and chicken is cooked through.

6. Chicken and Quinoa Salad:

Ingredients:
- 1 cup of cooked quinoa
- 1/2 cup of diced cooked chicken
- 1/2 cup of diced cucumber
- 1/2 cup of diced tomatoes
- 2 tablespoons of olive oil
- 1 tablespoon of lemon juice
- Salt and pepper to taste

Instructions:

1. In a bowl, combine the quinoa, chicken, cucumber, and tomatoes.
2. Drizzle the olive oil and lemon juice over the salad and mix to combine.
3. Season with salt and pepper to taste.
4. Serve and enjoy!

7. Tuna and Avocado Wrap:

Ingredients:

- 2 whole wheat tortillas
- 1/2 an avocado, mashed
- 1 can of tuna, drained
- 2 tablespoons of plain Greek yoghurt
- 1/4 cup of shredded carrots
- Salt and pepper to taste

Instructions:

1. Spread the mashed avocado onto the tortillas.
2. Top the tortillas with the tuna, Greek yoghurt, and shredded carrots.
3. Season with salt and pepper to taste.
4. Roll the tortillas into wraps and enjoy!

8. Turkey and Hummus Sandwich:

Ingredients:

- 2 slices of whole wheat bread
- 2 tablespoons of hummus
- 4 ounces of cooked turkey
- 1/4 cup of shredded lettuce
- 1/4 cup of diced tomato

Instructions:

1. Spread the hummus onto one side of the bread.
2. Top the bread with the turkey, lettuce, and tomato.
3. Place the other slice of bread on top and press down gently.
4. Cut the sandwich in half and enjoy!

9. Veggie Quesadilla:

Ingredients:
- 2 whole wheat tortillas
- 1/2 cup of shredded cheese
- 1/2 cup of diced bell peppers
- 1/4 cup of diced onion
- 2 tablespoons of olive oil

Instructions:

1. Heat the olive oil in a skillet over medium heat.
2. Add the bell peppers and onion and sauté for 3-4 minutes.
3. Place one of the tortillas into the skillet and top with the cheese and the bell pepper and onion mixture.
4. Place the other tortilla on top and cook for 3-4 minutes, or until the cheese has melted and the tortillas are golden brown.
5. Cut the quesadilla into slices and enjoy!

10. Lentil Soup:

Ingredients:

- 1 cup of lentils
- 2 cups of vegetable broth

- 1 cup of diced carrots
- 1 cup of diced celery
- 1/2 teaspoon of garlic powder
- Salt and pepper to taste

Instructions:

1. In a pot, combine the lentils, vegetable broth, carrots, celery, and garlic powder.
2. Bring the mixture to a boil over high heat.
3. Reduce the heat to low and simmer for 20 minutes, or until the lentils are tender.
4. Season with salt and pepper to taste.
5. Serve and enjoy!

11. Chickpea Salad Sandwich

Ingredients:

1 can chickpeas, drained and rinsed
2 tbsp tahini

2 tbsp lemon juice

1/4 cup chopped red onion

1/4 cup chopped celery

1/4 cup chopped dill pickles

Salt and pepper to taste

Whole grain bread

Instruction:

Mash chickpeas in a bowl using a fork. Add tahini, lemon juice, red onion, celery, dill pickles, salt, and pepper. Mix well. Spread chickpea salad on bread and top with your favourite sandwich toppings.

12. Greek Quinoa Salad

Ingredients:

1 cup cooked quinoa

1/2 cup cherry tomatoes, halved

1/2 cup diced cucumber

1/4 cup chopped red onion

1/4 cup crumbled feta cheese

2 tbsp lemon juice

1 tbsp olive oil

Salt and pepper to taste

Instruction:

In a large bowl, mix cooked quinoa, cherry tomatoes, cucumber, red onion, and feta cheese. In a small bowl, whisk together lemon juice, olive oil, salt, and pepper. Drizzle dressing over quinoa salad and toss to coat.

13. Turkey and Avocado Wrap

Ingredients:

whole wheat tortilla, roasted turkey breast, avocado, lettuce, tomato, red onion, hummus

Instructions:

Lay the tortilla flat on a plate. Spread hummus over the tortilla. Layer the turkey, avocado, lettuce, tomato, and red onion on top of the hummus. Roll up the tortilla tightly, tucking in the sides as you go. Slice in half and serve.

14. Quinoa Salad with Roasted Vegetables

Ingredients:

quinoa, mixed vegetables (such as bell peppers, zucchini, and eggplant), olive oil, salt, pepper, lemon juice, feta cheese

Instructions:

Cook quinoa according to package directions. Cut the mixed vegetables into bite-sized pieces and toss with olive oil, salt, and pepper. Roast in the oven at 400°F for 20-25 minutes, or until tender and golden brown. In a large bowl, combine the cooked quinoa and roasted vegetables. Drizzle with lemon juice and toss to combine. Crumble feta cheese over the top.

15. Chicken and Broccoli Stir-Fry

Ingredients:

boneless, skinless chicken breast, broccoli, garlic, soy sauce, oyster sauce, cornstarch, vegetable oil

Instructions:

Cut the chicken into bite-sized pieces. In a small bowl, whisk together soy sauce, oyster sauce, and cornstarch to make the sauce. Heat vegetable oil in a wok or large skillet over high heat. Add minced garlic and cook for 30 seconds, stirring constantly. Add the chicken and stir-fry until browned on all sides and cooked through about 5-7 minutes. Add broccoli and stir-fry for an additional 2-3 minutes, or until the broccoli is tender. Pour the sauce over the chicken and broccoli and stir-fry for 1-2 minutes, or until the sauce thickens.

16. Tuna Salad with Crackers

Ingredients:

canned tuna, celery, red onion, mayonnaise, Dijon mustard, lemon juice, salt, pepper, whole grain crackers

Instructions:

In a small bowl, combine canned tuna, finely chopped celery, and minced red onion. In a separate bowl, whisk together mayonnaise, Dijon mustard, lemon juice, salt, and pepper to make the dressing. Pour the dressing over the tuna mixture and stir to combine. Serve with whole-grain crackers.

17. Turkey and Hummus Wrap

Ingredients:

1 whole wheat wrap

3 slices of turkey breast

2 tbsp hummus

1/2 cup baby spinach leaves

1/4 cup sliced red bell pepper

1/4 cup sliced cucumber

Salt and pepper to taste

Instructions:

Lay the whole wheat wrap flat.

Spread hummus on the wrap.

Add turkey slices, spinach, red bell pepper, and cucumber.

Season with salt and pepper.

Roll the wrap tightly and slice it in half.

18. Quinoa Salad

Ingredients:
1 cup quinoa
1 can chickpeas, drained and rinsed
1/2 cup chopped fresh parsley
1/2 cup chopped fresh mint
1/4 cup chopped red onion
1/4 cup chopped cucumber
1/4 cup chopped tomato
2 tbsp olive oil
2 tbsp lemon juice

Salt and pepper to taste

Instructions:

Cook quinoa according to package instructions.

In a large bowl, combine cooked quinoa, chickpeas, parsley, mint, red onion, cucumber, and tomato.

Drizzle olive oil and lemon juice over the salad.

Season with salt and pepper to taste.

19. Tuna Salad Lettuce Wraps

Ingredients:

2 cans of tuna, drained

1/4 cup chopped celery

1/4 cup chopped red onion

1/4 cup chopped pickle

1/4 cup mayonnaise

2 tbsp Dijon mustard

1 tbsp lemon juice

Salt and pepper to taste

4-6 large lettuce leaves

Instructions:

In a bowl, mix the tuna, celery, red onion, and pickle.

In a separate bowl, whisk together the mayonnaise, Dijon mustard, and lemon juice.

Combine the mayonnaise mixture with the tuna mixture.

Season with salt and pepper to taste.

Spoon the tuna salad onto lettuce leaves and wrap them up.

20. Chickpea and Vegetable Curry

Ingredients:
1 tbsp olive oil
1 onion, chopped
2 garlic cloves, minced

1 tbsp curry powder

1/4 tsp turmeric

1 can chickpeas, drained and rinsed

1 can dice tomatoes

1 cup mixed vegetables (such as green beans, carrots, and peas)

Salt and pepper to taste

Instructions:

Heat olive oil in a large skillet over medium heat.

Add the onion and garlic and cook until softened.

Add curry powder and turmeric and cook for 1-2 minutes.

Add chickpeas, diced tomatoes, and mixed vegetables to the skillet.

21. Salmon and Asparagus Sheet Pan Dinner:

Ingredients:

- 2 salmon fillets
- 2 cups of asparagus spears
- 2 tablespoons of olive oil
- 1/2 teaspoon of garlic powder
- Salt and pepper to taste

Instructions:

1. Preheat the oven to 400°F.
2. Line a baking sheet with parchment paper.
3. Place the salmon fillets and asparagus spears onto the baking sheet.
4. Drizzle the olive oil over the salmon and asparagus and season with garlic powder, salt, and pepper.

5. Bake for 15-20 minutes, or until the salmon is cooked through and the asparagus is tender.

6. Serve and enjoy!

22. Pork Chops with Roasted Sweet Potatoes:

Ingredients:

- 2 pork chops
- 2 sweet potatoes, diced
- 2 tablespoons of olive oil
- 1 teaspoon of dried thyme
- Salt and pepper to taste

Instructions:

1. Preheat the oven to 400°F.
2. Line a baking sheet with parchment paper.

3. Place the pork chops and sweet potatoes onto the baking sheet.

4. Drizzle the olive oil over the pork chops and sweet potatoes and season with thyme, salt, and pepper.

5. Bake for 25-30 minutes, or until the pork chops are cooked through and the sweet potatoes are tender.

6. Serve and enjoy!

23. Chicken and Vegetable Stir-Fry:

Ingredients:

- 2 chicken breasts, diced
- 2 cups of broccoli florets
- 1/2 cup of diced bell peppers
- 2 tablespoons of olive oil
- 2 cloves of garlic, minced
- 2 tablespoons of soy sauce

Instructions:

1. Heat the olive oil in a large skillet over medium heat.
2. Add the diced chicken and cook for 4-5 minutes, or until cooked through.
3. Add the broccoli, bell peppers, garlic, and soy sauce and sauté for 3-4 minutes, or until the vegetables are tender.
3. Serve and enjoy!

24. Vegetarian Chili:

Ingredients:

- 1 can of black beans, rinsed and drained
- 1 can of kidney beans, rinsed and drained
- 1 can of diced tomatoes
- 1 cup of corn

- 1/2 cup of diced onion
- 2 tablespoons of chilli powder
- 1 teaspoon of cumin
- Salt and pepper to taste

Instructions:

1. In a pot, combine the black beans, kidney beans, diced tomatoes, corn, onion, chilli powder, and cumin.
2. Bring the mixture to a boil over high heat.
3. Reduce the heat to low and simmer for 15-20 minutes, or until the chilli has thickened.
4. Season with salt and pepper to taste.
5. Serve and enjoy!

25. Turkey and Zucchini Meatballs:

Ingredients:

- 1 pound of ground turkey
- 1/2 cup of grated zucchini
- 1/4 cup of minced onion
- 2 cloves of garlic, minced
- 2 tablespoons of olive oil
- 1 teaspoon of oregano
- Salt and pepper to taste

Instructions:

1. Preheat the oven to 375°F.
2. Line a baking sheet with parchment paper.
3. In a bowl, mix the ground turkey, zucchini, onion, garlic, oregano, salt, and pepper.

4. Form the mixture into small meatballs and place them onto

DINNER RECIPES:

1. Greek-Style Stuffed Peppers:
Ingredient:
4 bell peppers

1 lb lean ground turkey

1 cup cooked quinoa

1/2 onion diced

1/2 cup feta cheese

1/4 cup chopped fresh parsley

1 tsp dried oregano, salt and pepper to taste.

Instruction:
Preheat the oven to 375°F. Cut off the tops of the bell peppers and remove the seeds and membranes. In a skillet over

medium-high heat, cook the turkey and onion until the turkey is no longer pink. Add the cooked quinoa, feta cheese, parsley, oregano, salt, and pepper to the skillet and stir to combine. Fill each pepper with the turkey mixture and place in a baking dish. Cover the dish with foil and bake for 30 minutes. Remove the foil and bake for another 10 minutes, or until the peppers are tender.

2. One-Pan Balsamic Chicken and Vegetables:

Ingredients:

4 boneless

skinless chicken breasts

2 cups chopped broccoli

2 cups chopped cauliflower

1/2 red onion sliced

1/4 cup balsamic vinegar

2 tbsp olive oil

garlic cloves minced

1 tsp dried thyme

salt and pepper to taste.

Instruction:

Preheat the oven to 400°F. In a bowl, whisk together the balsamic vinegar, olive oil, garlic, thyme, salt, and pepper. Place the chicken breasts on one side of a baking sheet, and the chopped vegetables on the other. Drizzle the balsamic mixture over everything. Bake for 20-25 minutes, or until the chicken is cooked through and the vegetables are tender.

3. Spicy Thai Basil Shrimp:

Ingredients:

1 lb shrimp

peeled and deveined

2 tbsp oil

4 garlic cloves minced

1 red bell pepper sliced

1 yellow bell pepper sliced

1 onion sliced

2 tbsp oyster sauce

2 tbsp soy sauce

1 tsp sugar

1/2 cup Thai basil leaves.

Instruction:

In a wok or large skillet over high heat, add the oil and garlic and cook for 30 seconds. Add the shrimp and stir-fry for 1-2 minutes. Add the bell peppers and onion and stir-fry for another 2-3 minutes.

Add the oyster sauce, soy sauce, sugar, and Thai basil leaves and stir-fry for another minute, until everything is heated through.

4. Veggie-Packed Quinoa Bowl:
Ingredients:

1 cup cooked quinoa

1/2 cup diced sweet potato

1/2 cup sliced mushrooms

1/2 cup diced zucchini

1/2 cup diced bell pepper

2 cups baby spinach

1/4 cup crumbled feta cheese

1/4 cup chopped fresh parsley

2 tbsp olive oil

2 tbsp lemon juice

salt and pepper to taste.

Instruction:

In a skillet over medium-high heat, cook the sweet potato, mushrooms, zucchini, and bell pepper until tender. Add the baby spinach and cook until wilted. In a bowl, combine the cooked quinoa, cooked vegetables, feta cheese, and parsley. Drizzle with olive oil and lemon juice and season with salt and pepper.

5. Baked Salmon with Roasted Vegetables

Ingredients:

4 salmon fillets

1 lb. brussels sprouts, trimmed and halved

1 lb. sweet potatoes, peeled and diced

1 tbsp. olive oil

1 tsp. dried thyme

Salt and pepper to taste

Instructions:

Preheat the oven to 400°F.

Toss the brussels sprouts and sweet potatoes with olive oil, thyme, salt, and pepper. Arrange them on a baking sheet.

Place the salmon fillets on top of the vegetables.

Bake for 15-20 minutes, or until the salmon is cooked through and the vegetables are tender.

6. Turkey Chili

Ingredients:

1 lb. ground turkey

1 onion, chopped

2 cloves garlic, minced

1 red bell pepper, chopped

1 can (14 oz.) diced tomatoes

1 can (14 oz.) kidney beans, drained and rinsed

1 can (4 oz.) diced green chillies

1 tbsp. chilli powder

1 tsp. ground cumin

Salt and pepper to taste

Instructions:

In a large pot or Dutch oven, cook the ground turkey over medium-high heat until browned.

Add the onion, garlic, and red bell pepper and cook until softened.

Add the diced tomatoes, kidney beans, green chillies, chilli powder, cumin, salt, and pepper.

Bring the chilli to a simmer and cook for 20-30 minutes, stirring occasionally.

7. Stuffed Bell Peppers

Ingredients:

4 bell peppers, halved and seeded

1 lb. ground beef

1 onion, chopped

2 cloves garlic, minced

1 can (14 oz.) diced tomatoes

1 cup cooked rice

1 tsp. dried oregano

Salt and pepper to taste

Instructions:

Preheat the oven to 350°F.

In a large skillet, cook the ground beef over medium-high heat until browned.

Add the onion and garlic and cook until softened.

Stir in the diced tomatoes, cooked rice, oregano, salt, and pepper.

Fill the bell pepper halves with the beef mixture.

Place the stuffed peppers in a baking dish and cover with foil.

Bake for 25-30 minutes, or until the peppers are tender.

8. Grilled Chicken with Vegetables
Ingredients:

4 boneless, skinless chicken breasts

2 zucchini, sliced

1 yellow squash, sliced

1 red onion, sliced

1 red bell pepper, sliced

1/4 cup olive oil

1 tsp. dried basil

Salt and pepper to taste

Instructions:

Preheat the grill to medium-high heat.

In a large bowl, whisk together the olive oil, basil, salt, and pepper.

Add the chicken and vegetables to the bowl and toss to coat with the marinade.

Grill the chicken and vegetables for 10-12 minutes, or until the chicken is cooked through and the vegetables are tender.

9. Vegetarian Stuffed Bell Peppers
Ingredients:
4 large bell peppers, halved and seeded
1 cup cooked quinoa
1 cup canned black beans, rinsed and drained
1 cup canned corn, drained
1/2 cup diced red onion
1/2 cup diced tomato
1/2 cup shredded cheddar cheese
1 tablespoon olive oil
1 teaspoon chilli powder

1 teaspoon cumin

Salt and pepper, to taste

Instructions:

Preheat the oven to 375°F.

In a large bowl, combine the cooked quinoa, black beans, corn, red onion, tomato, olive oil, chilli powder, cumin, salt, and pepper.

Place the bell pepper halves in a baking dish and stuff each one with the quinoa and vegetable mixture.

Cover the baking dish with foil and bake for 35-40 minutes.

Remove the foil, sprinkle the shredded cheese on top of the stuffed peppers, and bake for an additional 10 minutes or until the cheese is melted and bubbly.

Serve hot and enjoy!

10. Baked Salmon with Roasted Broccoli:

Ingredients:

- 2 salmon fillets
- 2 cups of broccoli florets
- 2 tablespoons of olive oil
- 1/2 teaspoon of garlic powder
- Salt and pepper to taste

Instructions:

1. Preheat the oven to 400°F.
2. Line a baking sheet with parchment paper.
3. Place the salmon fillets and broccoli florets onto the baking sheet.
4. Drizzle the olive oil over the salmon and broccoli and season with garlic powder, salt, and pepper.

5. Bake for 15-20 minutes, or until the salmon is cooked through and the broccoli is tender.

6. Serve and enjoy!

11. Chicken Fajitas:

Ingredients:

- 2 chicken breasts, thinly sliced
- 1/2 cup of diced bell peppers
- 1/2 cup of diced onion
- 2 tablespoons of olive oil
- 1 teaspoon of cumin
- 1 teaspoon of chilli powder
- Salt and pepper to taste

Instructions:

1. Heat the olive oil in a large skillet over medium heat.

2. Add the chicken, bell peppers, and onion and sauté for 4-5 minutes.

3. Add the cumin, chilli powder, salt, and pepper and mix to combine.

4. Cook for an additional 3-4 minutes, or until the vegetables are tender.

5. Serve in warm tortillas and enjoy!

12. Veggie Burger:

Ingredients:

- 1 can of black beans, rinsed and drained
- 1/2 cup of cooked quinoa
- 1/2 cup of diced bell peppers
- 2 tablespoons of olive oil
- 2 cloves of garlic, minced
- 1/2 teaspoon of paprika
- Salt and pepper to taste

Instructions:

1. Heat the olive oil in a large skillet over medium heat.

2. Add the black beans, quinoa, bell peppers, garlic, paprika, salt, and pepper.

3. Mash the mixture with a potato masher and sauté for 3-4 minutes, or until the vegetables are tender.

4. Form the mixture into patties and cook for an additional 3-4 minutes, or until the patties are golden brown.

5. Serve and enjoy!

13. Turkey and Rice Casserole:

Ingredients:

- 2cups of cooked rice
- 2 cups of cooked turkey, diced
- 1 cup of diced bell peppers

- 1 cup of diced onion
- 1 can of diced tomatoes
- 2 tablespoons of olive oil
- 2 teaspoons of Italian seasoning
- Salt and pepper to taste

Instructions:

1. Preheat the oven to 375°F.
2. Heat the olive oil in a large skillet over medium heat.
3. Add the bell peppers and onion and sauté for 3-4 minutes.
4. In a large bowl, mix the cooked rice, turkey, diced tomatoes, bell pepper and onion mixture.
5. Add the Italian seasoning, salt, and pepper and mix to combine.
6. Transfer the mixture to an oven-safe dish and bake for 25-30 minutes, or until

the casserole is heated through and the top is golden brown.

7. Serve and enjoy!

14. Grilled Salmon with Sweet Potato Wedges and Asparagus

Ingredients:

4 salmon fillets

4 sweet potatoes, cut into wedges

1 bunch of asparagus

2 tbsp. olive oil

1 tbsp. garlic powder

Salt and pepper to taste

Instructions:

Preheat the grill to medium-high heat.

Toss sweet potato wedges with 1 tbsp. olive oil, garlic powder, salt, and pepper. Grill for 10-15 minutes or until tender.

Brush salmon fillets with 1 tbsp. olive oil and season with salt and pepper. Grill for 6-8 minutes on each side.

Toss asparagus with 1 tsp. olive oil and grill for 5-7 minutes.

Serve grilled salmon with sweet potato wedges and asparagus.

15. Chicken and Vegetable Stir Fry
Ingredients:
1 lb. boneless, skinless chicken breast, cut into thin strips
1 bell pepper, sliced
1 onion, sliced
1 cup broccoli florets
1 cup sliced carrots
2 tbsp. olive oil

1 tbsp. garlic, minced

Salt and pepper to taste

Instructions:

Heat 1 tbsp. olive oil in a large pan over medium-high heat. Add chicken and cook until browned on both sides.

Remove chicken from the pan and set aside.

Add remaining 1 tbsp. olive oil to the same pan. Add bell pepper, onion, broccoli, and carrots. Stir fry for 5-7 minutes or until vegetables is tender.

Add garlic to the pan and stir fry for 1-2 minutes.

Add chicken back to the pan and stir fry for 2-3 minutes.

Season with salt and pepper to taste.

Serve hot.

16. Baked Turkey Meatballs with Zucchini Noodles

Ingredients:

1 lb. ground turkey

1 egg

1/2 cup almond flour

1 tbsp. garlic powder

1 tbsp. dried oregano

1 tbsp. dried basil

Salt and pepper to taste

4 zucchinis, spiralized

1/4 cup chopped fresh parsley

1 tbsp. olive oil

1 cup marinara sauce

Instructions:

Preheat oven to 375°F. Line a baking sheet with parchment paper.

In a large bowl, mix ground turkey, egg, almond flour, garlic powder, oregano, basil, salt, and pepper.

Shape mixture into 16-18 meatballs.

Place meatballs on the prepared baking sheet and bake for 20-25 minutes, or until browned and cooked through.

Heat olive oil in a pan over medium heat. Add zucchini noodles and sauté for 3-5 minutes.

Add marinara sauce to the pan and stir until heated through.

Serve turkey meatballs with zucchini noodles and marinara sauce. Garnish with chopped parsley.

17. Stuffed Bell Peppers
Ingredients:
4 bell peppers, halved and seeded
1 lb. lean ground beef
1 cup cooked brown rice
1 onion, chopped
1 cup chopped mushrooms
2 garlic cloves, minced

1 tsp. chilli powder

Salt and pepper to taste

1 cup shredded cheddar cheese

Instructions:

Preheat oven to 375°F. Line a baking sheet with parchment paper

Sprinkle the remaining shredded cheese on top of each pepper.

Bake the stuffed peppers in the preheated oven for 25-30 minutes, or until the cheese is melted and bubbly and the peppers are tender.

Remove the peppers from the oven and allow them to cool for a few minutes before serving.

Garnish the peppers with chopped fresh parsley, if desired, and serve hot.

Enjoy your delicious and healthy stuffed bell peppers!

18. Grilled Lemon-Herb Chicken with Roasted Vegetables

Ingredients:

4 boneless, skinless chicken breasts

1/4 cup olive oil

3 tablespoons lemon juice

1 tablespoon chopped fresh herbs (such as thyme, rosemary, or oregano)

Salt and pepper to taste

2 cups mixed chopped vegetables (such as bell peppers, zucchini, and onions)

Instructions:

In a small bowl, whisk together the olive oil, lemon juice, chopped herbs, salt, and pepper.

Add the chicken breasts to the bowl and toss to coat in the marinade. Cover and refrigerate for at least 30 minutes, or up to 2 hours.

Preheat a grill or grill pan to medium-high heat.

Grill the chicken for 6-8 minutes per side, or until cooked through.

While the chicken is grilling, toss the chopped vegetables with a drizzle of olive oil, salt, and pepper.

Roast the vegetables in the oven at 400°F for 15-20 minutes, or until tender and slightly caramelized.

Serve the grilled chicken with the roasted vegetables on the side.

19. Spicy Shrimp Stir-Fry with Rice Noodles
Ingredients:

8 oz rice noodles

1 lb large shrimp, peeled and deveined

1 tablespoon olive oil

1 tablespoon grated fresh ginger

2 cloves garlic, minced

1 red bell pepper, thinly sliced

1 cup snow peas

1/4 cup soy sauce

1 tablespoon sriracha

1 tablespoon honey

2 tablespoons chopped fresh cilantro

Instructions:

Cook the rice noodles according to the package instructions. Drain and set aside.

Heat the olive oil in a large skillet or wok over high heat.

Add the shrimp and stir-fry for 2-3 minutes, or until pink and cooked through. Remove from the skillet and set aside.

Add the ginger and garlic to the skillet and stir-fry for 30 seconds.

Add the sliced bell pepper and snow peas to the skillet and stir-fry for 2-3 minutes, or until crisp-tender.

In a small bowl, whisk together the soy sauce, sriracha, and honey.

Add the cooked rice noodles and shrimp back to the skillet, along with the soy sauce mixture. Toss everything together and cook for 1-2 minutes, or until heated through.

Top the stir-fry with chopped cilantro and serve hot.

20. Baked Salmon with Asparagus and Quinoa

Ingredients:

4 salmon fillets

1 bunch of asparagus, trimmed

2 cups cooked quinoa

2 tablespoons olive oil

1 tablespoon Dijon mustard

1 tablespoon honey

1 tablespoon chopped fresh dill

Salt and pepper to taste

Instructions:

Preheat the oven to 400°F. Line a baking sheet with parchment paper.

Arrange the salmon fillets and asparagus on the baking sheet.

In a small bowl, whisk together the olive oil, Dijon mustard, honey, chopped dill, salt, and pepper.

Drizzle the sauce over the salmon and asparagus.

Bake in the preheated oven for 12-15 minutes, or until the salmon is cooked through and the asparagus is tender.

Serve the baked salmon and asparagus with the cooked quinoa on the side.

21. Lemon Garlic Butter Salmon:
Ingredients:
4 (6 oz) skinless salmon fillets
4 tbsp butter
2 garlic cloves, minced

2 tbsp fresh parsley, chopped

2 tbsp fresh lemon juice

Salt and pepper, to taste

Instructions:

Preheat oven to 400°F (200°C).

Melt butter in a saucepan over medium heat. Add minced garlic and cook until fragrant, about 1-2 minutes. Remove from heat.

Add chopped parsley and lemon juice to the garlic butter and mix well.

Place salmon fillets in a baking dish and season with salt and pepper.

Pour the garlic butter mixture over the salmon fillets, making sure they are well coated.

Bake in the oven for 10-12 minutes, or until salmon is cooked through.

21. Quinoa Stuffed Peppers:

Ingredients:

4 bell peppers, halved and seeded

1 cup quinoa, rinsed and drained

1 can black beans, rinsed and drained

1 can dice tomatoes, drained

1 cup frozen corn kernels

1 onion, diced

2 garlic cloves, minced

1 tsp chilli powder

1/2 tsp cumin

Salt and pepper, to taste

1/2 cup shredded cheddar cheese

Instructions:

Preheat oven to 350°F (175°C).

Cook quinoa according to package directions.

In a large skillet, sauté onion and garlic until translucent.

Add black beans, diced tomatoes, corn, chili powder, cumin, salt, and pepper to the skillet. Mix well and cook for a few minutes until heated through.

Add cooked quinoa to the skillet and mix well.

Place the bell pepper halves in a baking dish and fill each half with the quinoa and vegetable mixture.

Sprinkle shredded cheddar cheese on top of the stuffed peppers.

Bake in the oven for 20-25 minutes, or until the peppers are tender and the cheese is melted and bubbly.

SNACK RECIPES

here are five delicious snack recipes that are macro-friendly:

1. Apple Slices with Almond Butter

Ingredients:

1 medium apple

2 tbsp almond butter

Instructions:

Wash and slice the apple into thin wedges.

Spread the almond butter on each slice.

Serve and enjoy!

2. Chocolate Protein Balls

Ingredients:

1 cup rolled oats

1/2 cup chocolate protein powder

1/2 cup natural peanut butter

1/4 cup honey

Instructions:

In a bowl, mix the rolled oats and protein powder.

Add the peanut butter and honey and mix until well combined.

Roll the mixture into small balls.

Refrigerate for at least 30 minutes before serving.

3. Greek Yogurt Parfait

Ingredients:

1 cup plain Greek yoghurt

1/2 cup mixed berries
1/4 cup chopped nuts
1 tsp honey

Instructions:

In a glass or bowl, layer the Greek yoghurt, mixed berries, and chopped nuts.
Drizzle with honey.
Serve and enjoy!

4. Hummus with Vegetables

Ingredients:

1/2 cup hummus
1 cup sliced vegetables (such as carrots, cucumbers, and bell peppers)

Instructions:

Place the hummus in a small bowl.

Arrange the sliced vegetables around the hummus.

Serve and enjoy!

5. Turkey Roll-Ups

Ingredients:

4 slices deli turkey

4 slices Swiss cheese

1/2 cup baby spinach leaves

Instructions:

Lay a slice of turkey on a plate.

Place a slice of Swiss cheese on top.

Add a handful of baby spinach leaves.

Roll up tightly and slice into bite-size pieces.

Serve and enjoy!

6. Fruit and Nut Trail Mix:
Ingredients:
- 1/2 cup of almonds
- 1/2 cup of walnuts
- 1/2 cup of dried cranberries
- 1/2 cup of dried apricots

Instructions:
1. In a bowl, mix the almonds, walnuts, dried cranberries, and dried apricots.
2. Store in an airtight container and enjoy!

7. Avocado Toast:
Ingredients:
- 2 slices of whole wheat toast
- 1/2 an avocado, mashed
- 1 tablespoon of olive oil
- Salt and pepper to taste

Instructions:

1. Toast the two slices of whole wheat toast until golden brown.
2. Spread the mashed avocado onto the toast.
3. Drizzle the olive oil over the toast and season with salt and pepper to taste.
4. Enjoy!

8. Hummus and Veggie Sticks:
Ingredients:
- 1/2 cup of hummus
- 1/2 cup of carrots, cut into sticks
- 1/2 cup of celery, cut into sticks
- 1/2 cup of bell peppers, cut into sticks

Instructions:
1. Place the hummus in a bowl and arrange the carrot, celery, and bell pepper sticks around it.

2. Dip the vegetables into the hummus and enjoy!

9. Yogurt Parfait:
Ingredients:

- 1 cup of plain Greek yoghurt
- 1/2 cup of granola
- 1/4 cup of blueberries
- 1/4 cup of raspberries

Instructions:

1. In a bowl, layer the Greek yoghurt, granola, blueberries, and raspberries.
2. Mix to combine.
3. Enjoy!

10. Apple and Peanut Butter:
Ingredients:

- 1 apple, sliced
- 2 tablespoons of peanut butter

Instructions:

1. Spread the peanut butter onto the apple slices.
2. Enjoy!

11. Baked Sweet Potato Chips
Ingredients:

1 large sweet potato, washed and thinly sliced

1 tbsp olive oil

1/4 tsp sea salt

1/4 tsp smoked paprika

Preheat oven to 400°F. Toss sweet potato slices in olive oil, salt, and paprika. Spread out in a single layer on a baking sheet lined with parchment paper. Bake for 20-25 minutes or until crispy.

12. Chocolate Protein Balls

Ingredients:

1 cup rolled oats

1/2 cup chocolate protein powder

1/4 cup almond butter

1/4 cup honey

1/4 cup dark chocolate chips

Instructions:

Combine all ingredients in a bowl and mix well. Roll into bite-sized balls and chill in the fridge for at least 30 minutes.

13. Ants on a Log

Ingredients:

4 celery stalks, cut into 3-inch pieces

4 tbsp almond butter

1/4 cup raisins

Instructions:

Spread almond butter into each celery piece and top with raisins.

14. Fruit Salad with Yogurt

Ingredients:

1 cup mixed berries (strawberries, blueberries, raspberries)

1 cup diced pineapple

1 cup diced mango

1 cup plain Greek yoghurt

1 tbsp honey

Combine the fruit in a bowl. In a separate bowl, mix yoghurt and honey. Drizzle over fruit and serve.

15. Spiced Popcorn

Ingredients:

1/4 cup popcorn kernels

2 tbsp coconut oil

1/2 tsp chilli powder

1/2 tsp cumin

1/2 tsp garlic powder

Instructions:

Pop popcorn according to package instructions. Melt coconut oil in a small pan over low heat. Add chilli powder, cumin, and garlic powder and stir to combine. Drizzle over popcorn and toss to coat.

16. Greek Yogurt with Honey and Berries
Ingredients:

1 cup of Greek yoghurt

1 tablespoon of honey

1/2 cup of mixed berries (such as strawberries, blueberries, and raspberries)

Instructions:

In a bowl, mix the Greek yoghurt and honey.

Top with mixed berries and enjoy!

17. Spicy Roasted Chickpeas

Ingredients:

1 can of chickpeas, drained and rinsed

1 tablespoon of olive oil

1 teaspoon of paprika

1/2 teaspoon of cumin

1/2 teaspoon of garlic powder

1/4 teaspoon of cayenne pepper

Salt and pepper to taste

Instructions:

Preheat the oven to 400°F (200°C).

In a bowl, mix the chickpeas, olive oil, paprika, cumin, garlic powder, cayenne pepper, salt, and pepper.

Spread the chickpeas in a single layer on a baking sheet and bake for 20-25 minutes, or until crispy.

18. Apple Slices with Almond Butter

Ingredients:

1 apple, sliced

2 tablespoons of almond butter

Instructions:

Spread the almond butter on the apple slices.

Enjoy as a healthy and satisfying snack.

19. Cucumber and Hummus Bites

Ingredients:

1 cucumber, sliced

1/4 cup of hummus

1 tablespoon of chopped fresh parsley

Instructions:

Spread the hummus on the cucumber slices.

Sprinkle with chopped parsley.

Serve and enjoy!

20. Cottage Cheese with Tomato and Basil

Ingredients:

1/2 cup of cottage cheese

1/2 tomato, diced

2-3 fresh basil leaves, chopped

Salt and pepper to taste

Instructions:

In a bowl, mix the cottage cheese, diced tomato, chopped basil, salt, and pepper.

Enjoy as a healthy and refreshing snack.

21. Roasted Chickpeas

Ingredients:

1 can chickpeas, drained and rinsed

1 tbsp olive oil

1 tsp paprika

1/2 tsp cumin

1/2 tsp garlic powder

Salt to taste

Instructions:

Preheat the oven to 400°F (200°C). Pat the chickpeas dry with a paper towel, then toss with olive oil, paprika, cumin, garlic powder, and salt. Spread the chickpeas out in a single layer on a baking sheet and bake for 20-25 minutes, stirring occasionally, until crispy and golden brown.

22. Yogurt Parfait
Ingredients:
1/2 cup plain Greek yoghurt
1/4 cup granola
1/2 cup mixed berries

Layer the yoghurt, granola, and mixed berries in a tall glass or jar. Repeat the layers until all the ingredients are used up.

23. Apple Slices with Almond Butter

Ingredients:

1 apple, sliced

2 tbsp almond butter

Cinnamon to taste

Instructions:

Spread the almond butter on the apple slices and sprinkle with cinnamon. Enjoy as a healthy and satisfying snack.

DESSERT RECIPES

here are some macro-friendly dessert recipes:

1. Chocolate Protein Mug Cake

Ingredients:

1 scoop of chocolate protein powder

1 tbsp coconut flour

1 tbsp unsweetened cocoa powder

1/4 tsp baking powder

1 egg

1/4 cup unsweetened almond milk

1/2 tsp vanilla extract

1-2 packets of stevia (optional)

1 tbsp sugar-free chocolate chips (optional)

Instructions:

In a microwave-safe mug, mix the protein powder, coconut flour, cocoa powder, and baking powder.

Add the egg, almond milk, vanilla extract, and stevia (if using) to the mug and stir well.

Stir in the chocolate chips (if using).

Microwave the mug on high for 60-90 seconds, or until the cake has risen and is set in the centre.

Let the cake cool for a few minutes before enjoying it.

2. Banana Oat Cookies

Ingredients:

2 ripe bananas, mashed

1 cup rolled oats

1/2 tsp cinnamon

1/4 tsp salt

1/4 cup chopped walnuts (optional)

Instructions:

Preheat the oven to 350°F (180°C) and line a baking sheet with parchment paper.

In a mixing bowl, combine the mashed bananas, oats, cinnamon, and salt.

Stir in the chopped walnuts (if using).

Scoop the mixture onto the prepared baking sheet, using a spoon or cookie scoop to form cookie shapes.

Bake for 15-20 minutes, or until the cookies are lightly browned and set.

Let the cookies cool before enjoying them.

3. Peanut Butter Protein Balls
Ingredients:

1 cup rolled oats

1/2 cup natural peanut butter

1/4 cup honey or maple syrup

1 scoop vanilla protein powder

1/4 cup mini chocolate chips (optional)

Instructions:

In a mixing bowl, combine the oats, peanut butter, honey or maple syrup, and protein powder.

Stir in the chocolate chips (if using).

Use your hands to roll the mixture into bite-sized balls.

Place the balls on a baking sheet lined with parchment paper and refrigerate for at least 30 minutes to set.

Once the balls are set, they can be stored in an airtight container in the refrigerator for up to one week.

4. Chocolate Chip Cookies:

Ingredients:

- 1 cup of butter, softened
- 1 cup of brown sugar
- 1 cup of granulated sugar

- 2 eggs

- 2 teaspoons of vanilla extract

- 2 1/2 cups of all-purpose flour

- 1 teaspoon of baking soda

- 1 teaspoon of salt

- 2 cups of semisweet chocolate chips

Instructions:

1. Preheat the oven to 375°F.
2. In a large bowl, cream together the butter and sugars until light and fluffy.
3. Add the eggs and vanilla extract and mix to combine.
4. In a separate bowl, mix the flour, baking soda, and salt.
5. Slowly add the dry ingredients to the wet ingredients and mix until combined.
6. Fold in the chocolate chips.

7. Drop the cookie dough onto a baking sheet, about 2 inches apart.

8. Bake for 8-10 minutes, or until the cookies are golden brown.

9. Let's cool and enjoy!

5. Chocolate Brownies:

Ingredients:

- 1 cup of butter, melted

- 2 cups of sugar

- 4 eggs

- 1 1/2 cups of all-purpose flour

- 3/4 cup of cocoa powder

- 1 teaspoon of baking powder

- 1 teaspoon of salt

- 1 cup of semisweet chocolate chips

Instructions:

1. Preheat the oven to 350°F.

2. In a large bowl, mix the melted butter and sugar until combined.

3. Add the eggs and mix to combine.

4. In a separate bowl, mix the flour, cocoa powder, baking powder, and salt.

5. Slowly add the dry ingredients to the wet ingredients and mix until combined.

6. Fold in the chocolate chips.

7. Pour the mixture into a greased 9x13-inch baking pan and spread evenly.

8. Bake for 25-30 minutes, or until a toothpick inserted into the centre comes out clean.

9. Let's cool and enjoy!

6. Cheesecake:

Ingredients:

- 2 packages of cream cheese, softened
- 1/2 cup of sugar

- 2 eggs

- 1 teaspoon of vanilla extract

- 1/4 teaspoon of salt

- 1 prepared graham cracker crust

Instructions:

1. Preheat the oven to 325°F.
2. In a large bowl, cream together the cream cheese and sugar until light and fluffy.
3. Add the eggs, vanilla extract, and salt and mix to combine.
4. Pour the mixture into the prepared graham cracker crust.
5. Bake for 40-45 minutes, or until the centre is set.
6. Let's cool and enjoy!

7. Apple Crisp:

Ingredients:

- 4 apples, peeled and sliced
- 1/2 cup of brown sugar
- 1/2 cup of all-purpose flour
- 1/4 cup of butter, melted
- 1 teaspoon of cinnamon
- 1/2 teaspoon of nutmeg

Instructions:

1. Preheat the oven to 350°F.
2. Place the sliced apples into a 9x13-inch baking pan.
3. In a bowl, mix the brown sugar, flour, melted butter, cinnamon, and nutmeg.
4. Sprinkle the mixture over the apples.
5. Bake for 30-35 minutes, or until the top is golden brown.
6. Serve warm and enjoy!

8. Chocolate Avocado Pudding

Ingredients:

1 ripe avocado

1/4 cup unsweetened cocoa powder

1/4 cup pure maple syrup

1/4 cup almond milk

1 tsp vanilla extract

Pinch of salt

Optional toppings: chopped nuts, sliced banana, raspberries

Instructions:

In a food processor, blend avocado until smooth.

Add cocoa powder, maple syrup, almond milk, vanilla extract, and salt, and blend until well combined and smooth.

Transfer to a bowl and refrigerate for at least 1 hour.

Serve chilled with desired toppings.

9. Protein Brownies

Ingredients:

2 scoops chocolate protein powder

1/2 cup almond flour

1/2 cup unsweetened cocoa powder

1/2 cup unsweetened applesauce

1/4 cup pure maple syrup

1/4 cup almond milk

2 eggs

1 tsp vanilla extract

1/2 tsp baking powder

Pinch of salt

Instructions:

Preheat oven to 350°F.

In a large bowl, combine protein powder, almond flour, cocoa powder, baking powder, and salt.

In a separate bowl, whisk together applesauce, maple syrup, almond milk, eggs, and vanilla extract.

Add wet ingredients to dry ingredients and mix until well combined.

Pour batter into a greased 8x8-inch baking dish.

Bake for 20-25 minutes, or until a toothpick inserted into the centre comes out clean.

Let cool before cutting into squares.

10. Lemon Chia Seed Muffins
Ingredients:

2 cups almond flour

1/4 cup chia seeds

1/4 cup pure maple syrup

1/4 cup coconut oil, melted

3 eggs

1 tsp baking powder

1/2 tsp baking soda

1/2 tsp salt

Zest and juice of 2 lemons

11. Chocolate Peanut Butter Protein Balls

Ingredients:

1 cup old-fashioned oats

1/2 cup natural peanut butter

1/3 cup honey

1 scoop of chocolate protein powder

1/4 cup mini chocolate chips

Instructions:

In a mixing bowl, combine all ingredients except for the chocolate chips.

Mix until all ingredients are well combined.

Add in the chocolate chips and stir.

Roll the mixture into bite-sized balls.

Place in the fridge for at least 30 minutes before serving.

12. Banana Oat Cookies

Ingredients:

2 ripe bananas

1 cup old-fashioned oats

1/4 cup chocolate chips

1/4 cup chopped nuts (optional)

Instructions:

Preheat the oven to 350°F (175°C).

In a mixing bowl, mash the bananas until smooth.

Add in the oats and mix until well combined.

Stir in the chocolate chips and nuts (if using).

Drop spoonfuls of the mixture onto a baking sheet lined with parchment paper.

Bake for 15-20 minutes or until the cookies are lightly browned.

Let cool before serving.

13. Blueberry Protein Muffins
Ingredients:
1 cup almond flour
1 scoop vanilla protein powder
1/2 tsp baking powder
1/4 tsp salt
2 eggs

1/2 cup unsweetened almond milk

1/4 cup honey

1 tsp vanilla extract

1/2 cup fresh blueberries

Instructions:

Preheat the oven to 350°F (175°C) and line a muffin tin with liners.

In a mixing bowl, combine the almond flour, protein powder, baking powder, and salt.

In a separate bowl, whisk together the eggs, almond milk, honey, and vanilla extract.

Add the wet ingredients to the dry ingredients and mix until well combined.

Fold in the blueberries.

Divide the batter evenly among the muffin cups.

Bake for 18-20 minutes or until a toothpick inserted into the centre comes out clean.

Let cool before serving.

14. Chocolate Chia Pudding

Ingredients:

1/4 cup chia seeds

1 cup unsweetened almond milk

1 tbsp unsweetened cocoa powder

1 tbsp honey

1/4 tsp vanilla extract

In a mixing bowl, whisk together the chia seeds, almond milk, cocoa powder, honey, and vanilla extract.

Let the mixture sit for 5 minutes, then whisk again.

Cover the bowl and refrigerate for at least 2 hours or overnight.

Serve chilled, topped with fresh fruit or nuts if desired.

15. Apple Cinnamon Baked Oatmeal
Ingredients:
2 cups old-fashioned oats
1 tsp baking powder
1/2 tsp cinnamon
1/4 tsp salt

2 cups unsweetened almond milk

1/4 cup honey

1 tsp vanilla extract

1 apple, peeled and diced

1/4 cup chopped nuts (optional)

Instructions:

Preheat the oven to 375°F (190°C) and grease a baking dish.

In a mixing bowl, combine the oats, baking powder, cinnamon, and salt.

In a separate bowl, whisk together the almond milk, honey, and vanilla extract. Add the wet

16. Chocolate Protein Brownies

Ingredients:

1/2 cup almond flour

1/4 cup chocolate protein powder

1/4 cup unsweetened cocoa powder

1/4 cup honey

1/4 cup unsweetened almond milk

1/4 cup unsweetened applesauce

2 eggs

1 tsp vanilla extract

1/2 tsp baking powder

Pinch of salt

Instructions:

Preheat oven to 350°F.

In a large bowl, mix almond flour, protein powder, cocoa powder, baking powder, and salt.

In a separate bowl, whisk together honey, almond milk, applesauce, eggs, and vanilla extract.

Add wet ingredients to dry ingredients and stir until well combined.

Pour batter into a greased 8x8 inch baking dish and bake for 20-25 minutes, or until a toothpick comes out clean.

17. Peanut Butter Banana Oat Cookies
Ingredients:
2 ripe bananas, mashed
1/2 cup creamy peanut butter
1/4 cup honey
2 cups rolled oats
1 tsp vanilla extract
1/2 tsp ground cinnamon

Instructions:

Preheat oven to 350°F.

In a large bowl, mix mashed bananas, peanut butter, honey, vanilla extract, and cinnamon.

Add rolled oats to the bowl and stir until well combined.

Using a cookie scoop, drop the dough onto a parchment-lined baking sheet.

Bake for 12-15 minutes, or until the cookies are lightly browned.

18. Chocolate Chip Banana Bread
Ingredient:

2 ripe bananas, mashed

2 eggs

1/4 cup honey

1/4 cup unsweetened applesauce

1 tsp vanilla extract

1 3/4 cups almond flour

1 tsp baking powder

1/2 tsp baking soda

1/4 tsp salt

1/2 cup dark chocolate chips

Instructions:

Preheat oven to 350°F and grease a 9x5 inch loaf pan.

In a large bowl, whisk together mashed bananas, eggs, honey, applesauce, and vanilla extract.

In a separate bowl, mix almond flour, baking powder, baking soda, and salt.

Add dry ingredients to wet ingredients and stir until well combined.

Fold in chocolate chips.

Pour batter into prepared loaf pan and bake for 45-50 minutes, or until a toothpick comes out clean.

19. Berry Chia Pudding

Ingredients:

1 cup unsweetened almond milk

1/4 cup chia seeds

1/2 tsp vanilla extract

1/2 cup mixed berries

1 tbsp honey

Instructions:

In a jar or bowl, mix almond milk, chia seeds, and vanilla extract.

Cover and refrigerate for at least 2 hours or overnight.

In a separate bowl, mash mixed berries with honey.

Layer chia pudding and berry mixture in a serving glass or jar.

Serve chilled.

20. Cinnamon Apple Chips

Ingredients:

2 apples, thinly sliced

1 tbsp honey

1 tsp ground cinnamon

Instructions:

Preheat oven to 200°F.

In a small bowl, whisk together honey and cinnamon.

Arrange apple slices in a single layer on a parchment-lined baking sheet.

Brush apple slices with honey-cinnamon

21. Chocolate Chia Pudding:

Ingredients:

1/4 cup chia seeds

1 cup unsweetened almond milk

1 tablespoon unsweetened cocoa powder

1 tablespoon honey

1/2 teaspoon vanilla extract

Instructions:

In a small bowl, whisk together the chia seeds and almond milk. Add in the cocoa powder, honey, and vanilla extract and whisk until well combined. Cover and refrigerate for at least 2 hours or overnight. Serve chilled.

22. Almond Butter and Banana Bites:

Ingredients:

1 banana, sliced

2 tablespoons almond butter

2 tablespoons granola

Instructions:

Spread a small amount of almond butter onto each banana slice. Sprinkle with granola and serve.

23. Baked Apple with Cinnamon:

Ingredients:

1 apple, cored and sliced

1/2 teaspoon cinnamon

1 teaspoon honey

Instructions:

Preheat the oven to 350°F (175°C). Place the sliced apple on a baking sheet and sprinkle with cinnamon. Drizzle with honey and bake for 15-20 minutes, or until the apple is soft and slightly caramelized. Serve warm.

24. Chocolate Avocado Pudding:

Ingredients:

1 avocado, peeled and pitted

1/4 cup unsweetened almond milk

1/4 cup unsweetened cocoa powder

2 tablespoons honey

1/2 teaspoon vanilla extract

Instructions:

In a blender or food processor, combine the avocado, almond milk, cocoa powder, honey, and vanilla extract. Blend until smooth and creamy. Transfer to a bowl or individual serving dishes and refrigerate for at least 30 minutes before serving.

25. Coconut and Berry Chia Seed Pudding:

Ingredients:

1/4 cup chia seeds

1 cup unsweetened coconut milk

1 tablespoon honey

1/2 teaspoon vanilla extract

1/4 cup mixed berries

Instructions:

In a small bowl, whisk together the chia seeds and coconut milk. Add in the honey and vanilla extract and whisk until well combined. Cover and refrigerate for at least 2 hours or overnight. Top with mixed berries before serving.

CHAPTER SEVEN

STAYING ON TRACK WITH THE MACRO DIET

Tips for Dining Out

Following a macro diet doesn't mean you can't enjoy eating out at restaurants with friends and family. Here are some tips to help you make healthy choices when dining out:

Check the menu in advance: Look up the restaurant's menu online before going out to eat. This will help you plan and choose the healthiest options available.

Focus on protein: Aim to order dishes that include a good source of protein, such as grilled chicken, fish, or tofu. This will help keep you full and satisfied while also supporting muscle growth and repair.

Watch portion sizes: Restaurants often serve large portions that can easily derail your diet. Try to split an entrée with a friend, or ask for a to-go box and pack up half of your meal before you start eating.

Avoid creamy sauces and dressings: Sauces and dressings can be high in calories and fat. Opt for simple dishes that are grilled, baked, or steamed, and choose dressings on the side so you can control the amount you use.

Choose complex carbohydrates: When ordering carbs, choose complex carbohydrates like brown rice, sweet potatoes, or whole-grain bread instead of refined carbs like white rice or pasta.

Don't be afraid to ask for modifications: Many restaurants are willing to make substitutions or modifications to dishes to make them healthier. For example, ask for extra vegetables instead of french fries or a side salad instead of a baked potato.

Avoid sugary drinks: Many drinks, including soda and sweetened tea, are high in sugar and can quickly add up in calories. Stick with water or unsweetened tea to keep your calorie intake in check.

By following these tips, you can still enjoy eating out while staying on track with your macro diet and health goals.

Healthy Snacking Ideas

If you're looking for healthy snacking ideas to incorporate into your macro diet, here are a few options:

Fresh fruit: Opt for seasonal fruits like berries, apples, or oranges. Pair with some nut butter or Greek yoghurt for some extra protein.

Veggies and hummus: Cut up some veggies like carrots, cucumbers, or bell peppers and pair them with your favourite flavour of hummus.

Roasted chickpeas: Toss some chickpeas with olive oil and your favourite spices and roast them in the oven until they're crispy.

Hard-boiled eggs: Boil a batch of eggs at the beginning of the week and keep them on hand for a quick protein-packed snack.

Homemade trail mix: Mix some nuts, seeds, and dried fruit for a portable and filling snack.

Cottage cheese: Pair cottage cheese with fresh fruit or mix in some nuts and seeds for a filling and protein-packed snack.

Rice cakes with avocado and smoked salmon: Top a rice cake with mashed avocado and smoked salmon for a protein-rich and satisfying snack.

Edamame: Steam a batch of edamame and sprinkle it with sea salt for a protein-rich snack.

Greek yoghurt: Mix in some fresh fruit or granola for a protein-rich and satisfying snack.

Turkey roll-ups: Roll up turkey slices with some hummus, avocado, or veggies for a protein-rich and portable snack.

How to Handle Cravings

Handling cravings can be challenging, but it is an important part of maintaining a healthy and sustainable diet. Here are some tips for handling cravings:

Understand the reason behind the craving: Sometimes, cravings are simply the result of hunger, but they can also be triggered by stress, boredom, or emotions. Understanding the reason behind the craving can help you determine the best way to deal with it.

Keep healthy snacks on hand: Having healthy snacks on hand, such as fresh fruit, nuts, or raw vegetables, can help you resist the temptation to reach for less healthy options.

Practice mindfulness: Mindfulness techniques, such as deep breathing or meditation, can help you manage cravings by bringing awareness to the present moment and reducing stress and anxiety.

Find healthy alternatives: If you are craving a specific food, try to find a healthier alternative. For example, if you are craving something sweet, try a piece of fruit or a small serving of dark chocolate.

Allow yourself an occasional treat: It is okay to indulge in your favourite foods once in a while. Just be sure to enjoy them in moderation and balance them out with healthier choices.

Remember, handling cravings is not about denying yourself the foods you enjoy, but rather finding a balance between indulgence and healthy choices.

Staying Motivated

Staying motivated is an important part of any healthy lifestyle, including following a macro diet. Here are some tips for staying motivated:

Set Realistic Goals: Setting realistic and achievable goals will keep you motivated. Instead of focusing on losing 20 pounds in a month, set a goal of losing

1-2 pounds a week. This will give you a sense of accomplishment and motivate you to keep going.

Find a Support System: Having a support system can be very helpful in staying motivated. This can be a friend, family member, or even an online support group. You can share your progress, ask for advice, and get encouragement when you need it.

Reward Yourself: It's important to reward yourself for your progress. This doesn't have to be anything big, but something that will make you feel good. This could be a new workout outfit, a massage, or even a cheat meal.

Keep a Positive Attitude: A positive attitude is essential for staying motivated. Instead of focusing on what you can't eat, focus on what you can eat. Celebrate small victories and don't beat yourself up over setbacks.

Track Your Progress: Tracking your progress can help you stay motivated. This can be done through a food journal, taking progress pictures, or even using a fitness app. Seeing how far you've come can give you the motivation to keep going.

Mix Things Up: Doing the same thing every day can get boring. Mix up your workouts, try new recipes, and experiment with different foods. This will keep things interesting and help you stay motivated.

By following these tips, you can stay motivated on your macro diet journey and achieve your health and fitness goals.

CONCLUSION

Appendix: Macro Diet Food List Cheat Sheet

Here's a quick macro diet food list cheat sheet to help you when you're meal planning and grocery shopping:

Protein:

Chicken breast

Turkey breast

Lean beef (e.g. sirloin, tenderloin)

Pork loin

Fish (e.g. salmon, tilapia, tuna)

Shrimp

Tofu

Tempeh

Edamame

Greek yoghurt

Cottage cheese

Whey protein powder

Casein protein powder

Carbohydrates:
Brown rice
Quinoa
Whole wheat bread
Whole wheat pasta
Sweet potato
Oatmeal
Barley
Bulgur
Corn
Beans (e.g. black beans, chickpeas, kidney beans)
Lentils
Fruits (e.g. apples, bananas, berries, oranges, kiwi)
Vegetables (e.g. broccoli, spinach, carrots, bell peppers, tomatoes)

Fats:

Olive oil

Avocado

Almonds

Walnuts

Cashews

Peanut butter

Flaxseed oil

Chia seeds

Sesame seeds

Cheese (e.g. cheddar, mozzarella, feta)

Whole eggs

Egg yolks

Remember to always track your macros and calories to ensure you're meeting your nutritional goals.

You may easily and quickly refer to a Macro Diet Food List Cheat Sheet to help you stick to your macro diet plan. Here are some pointers on how to utilize it successfully:

Know your macros: Before using the cheat sheet, it's crucial to be aware of your daily macro objectives for protein, carbohydrates, and fats. This will assist you in picking the appropriate meals and serving sizes to adhere to your macro objectives.

Use portion sizes: The cheat sheet lists popular macro-friendly meals along with the amount of each nutrient in a serving.

To keep within your daily targets, make sure to measure or weigh your meals.

Choose whole foods: Even though the cheat sheet includes some processed items, it is typically preferable to pick full, nutrient-dense foods for optimum health and satisfaction.

Schedule your meals: To avoid having to make decisions on the spot, use the cheat sheet to schedule your meals and snacks in advance. This might assist you to avoid making hasty decisions that can mess up your macros.

Be adaptable: While it's crucial to adhere to your macro objectives, it's also crucial to be adaptable and not worry too much if you slightly go over or under. Keep in mind that progress, not perfection, is the goal.

You may choose nutritious foods and adhere to your macro objectives by utilizing the Macro Diet Food List Cheat Sheet as a reference.

References

Helms, E. R., Aragon, A. A., & Fitschen, P. J. (2014). Evidence-based recommendations for natural bodybuilding contest preparation: nutrition and supplementation. Journal of the International Society of Sports Nutrition, 11(1), 20.

Phillips, S. M., & Van Loon, L. J. (2011). Dietary protein for athletes: from requirements to optimum adaptation. Journal of sports sciences, 29(sup1), S29-S38.

Schoenfeld, B. J., Aragon, A. A., & Krieger, J. W. (2013). The effect of protein timing on muscle strength and hypertrophy: a meta-analysis. Journal of the

International Society of Sports Nutrition, 10(1), 53.

Tipton, K. D., & Witard, O. C. (2007). Protein requirements and recommendations for athletes: relevance of ivory tower arguments for practical recommendations. Clinical Nutrition, 26(2), 128-138.

Volek, J. S., & Rawson, E. S. (2004). Scientific basis and practical aspects of creatine supplementation for athletes. Nutrition, 20(7-8), 609-614.

Williams, M. H. (2005). Dietary supplements and sports performance: amino acids. Journal of the International Society of Sports Nutrition, 2(2), 63.

Wilson, J. M., Wilson, G. J., & Zourdos, M. C. (2012). Contemporary issues in protein requirements and consumption for resistance-trained athletes. Journal of the International Society of Sports Nutrition, 9(1), 5.

Index

Introduction

What is the Macro Diet?

How the Macro Diet Works

Benefits of the Macro Diet

Macros and Their Role in the Diet (Proteins, Carbohydrates, Fats)

Macro-Friendly Foods

Foods to Avoid

Grocery Shopping Tips

Creating a Meal Plan

Meal Planning Tips and Tricks

Prepping Meals in Advance

Healthy Cooking Techniques

Macro Diet Cooking Tips and Tricks

Breakfast Recipes

Lunch Recipes

Dinner Recipes

Snack Recipes

Dessert Recipes

Tips for Dining Out

Healthy Snacking Ideas

How to Handle Cravings

Staying Motivated

Macro Diet Food List Cheat Sheet

References

Printed in Great Britain
by Amazon